"A much-needed work, exploring the psychology of toilet functions on many levels: physical, psychological, social. At a time when many feel the world turning into a huge toilet in which all kinds of attitudes and emotions are being evacuated via war and group tensions, a serious exploration of individual and social evacuation functions could not be more welcome. This work examines many examples of urinary-defecation problems throughout a lifetime coupled with keen, pertinent clinical work and suggestions. Psychic toilets, world toilets, ordinary physical toilets and their difficulties are brought into focus with fresh acumen in ways aimed to help, challenge, and enrich."

Michael Eigen, PhD; *author, The Challenge of Being Human, The Sensitive Self, and Contact with the Depth*

.

Psychoanalysis and Toileting

Psychoanalysis and Toileting is an accessible book that delineates and interprets the psychological meanings of defecating and urinating in everyday life.

Paul Marcus' work gives the clinician an in-depth view of an activity that every patient and practitioner engage in and shows how not dealing with toileting in its wide range of social and practical contexts leaves out a huge aspect of the patient's everyday experience. Drawing from psychoanalytic theory and practice, the author discusses such subjects as constipation, diarrhea and irritable bowel syndrome, adult female incontinence, toilet cursing, public toilet graffiti and toilet humor. The book also considers the personal meaning of urinating and defecating as seen in men suffering from an enlarged prostate, in 'excremental assault' in the Nazi concentration camps, and in dreaming. Marcus considers not only what is typically negative about these experiences, but what can be seen as positive in terms of growth and development for the ordinary person. The book is illustrated throughout with clinical vignettes and observations taken from the author's private practice.

Psychoanalysis and Toileting will be a key text for psychoanalysts and psychoanalytic psychotherapists in practice and in training. It will also be relevant to other mental health practitioners.

Paul Marcus is a training and supervisory analyst at the National Psychological Association for Psychoanalysis in New York City and Co-Chairperson of the discussion group Psychoanalysis and Spirituality at the American Psychoanalytic Association.

Psychoanalysis and Toileting

Minding One's Business

Paul Marcus

Routledge
Taylor & Francis Group
LONDON AND NEW YORK

Designed cover image: Getty

First published 2023
by Routledge
4 Park Square, Milton Park, Abingdon, Oxon OX14 4RN

and by Routledge
605 Third Avenue, New York, NY 10158

Routledge is an imprint of the Taylor & Francis Group, an informa business

© 2023 Paul Marcus

British Library Cataloguing in Publication Data
A catalogue record for this book is available from the British Library

Library of Congress Cataloging-in-Publication Data
A catalog record has been requested for this book

ISBN: 9781032113937 (hbk)
ISBN: 9781032113951 (pbk)
ISBN: 9781003219705 (ebk)

DOI: 10.4324/9781003219705

Typeset in Times New Roman
by Taylor & Francis Books

Dedicated to Samuel L. Pauker, M.D. A great friend and a brilliant psychiatrist/psychoanalyst

Contents

Recently published Routledge titles by Paul Marcus

Psychoanalysis as a Spiritual Discipline. In Dialogue with Martin Buber and Gabriel Marcel (2021).

Psychoanalysis, Classic Social Psychology and Moral Living. Let the Conversation Begin (2020).

The Psychoanalysis of Overcoming Suffering. Flourishing Despite Pain (2019).

The Psychoanalysis of Career Choice, Job Performance, and Satisfaction. How to Flourish in the Workplace (2017).

Chapter 1

Introduction: Psychoanalysis and the Toilet

According to Freud's lifelong friend, colleague and biographer Ernest Jones, for at least "twenty years of his early manhood," Freud suffered from "severe indigestion, often with constipation, the functional nature of which he did not then recognize, and moodiness in pronounced degree.... that were of psychological origin" (sometimes distressingly mentioned in his letters to friends) (Jones, 1961, p. 114).[1] Moreover, in September 1909, notwithstanding Freud's travel phobia, he, Jung and Ferenczi engaged in a highly productive visit to America, though "Freud complained for the rest of his life about how American toilets ruined his bladder" (Kaplan, 2010, p. 206). Perhaps in part for these personal physical problems in everyday living, Freud wrote in a foreword to *Scatologica Rites of All Nations*, a fascinating 1891 ethnographic study of excrements by self-educated anthropologist/ Captain of the U.S. Third Cavalry, John Bourke, that "to make [the role of excretions in human life] more accessible... is not only a courageous but also a meritorious undertaking" (Freud, 1913, p. 9). Freud also wrote elsewhere in the same foreword, that it would be a "wiser course undoubtedly" for humanity "to admit its [excrements'] existence and dignify it as much as nature will allow" (ibid., p. 6). Indeed, as Eigen points out, "for some time, he [Freud] was particularly taken with shitting and wondered about the need to evacuate, which Freud also associated with creativity and making, as well as self-hate" (Eigen, 2022, p. 91).

While the act of going to the toilet is an everyday one that is intimately fused with our bodies (e.g., physical satisfaction, the appearance of cleanliness and bodily protocol), our senses (e.g. vision, smell, hearing/"aural privacy")[2] and our emotions (e.g. shame, embarrassment, anxiety, fear, disgust and desire), there has been a remarkable paucity of scholarly toilet studies. In fact, there are no psychoanalytic studies of the toilet as a subject, "and so little" of such studies in other disciplines

DOI: 10.4324/9781003219705-1

such as sociology and anthropology (Molotch, 2010, p. 18). That is, "toilet culture in general, and public necessities in particular, have rarely been considered worthy topics of study" (George, 2008, p. 134). As Barbara Penner, a prominent architectural historian, and one of the pioneers in toilet studies (especially as it relates to gender) noted, "Every discipline [is] constituted by what it forbids its practitioners to do" (she is quoting H. White's *Tropics of Discourse*), though in the case of toilet studies it is more pertinent to say, "by what it forbids its prac- titioners to speak about," including how it permits them to speak (Penner, 2010, p. 229). A similar sentiment was expressed by a promi- nent analyst, Salman Akhtar, "Cultural abhorrence of anal matters perhaps also adds to the 'heuristic repression' of the anal phase" (Akhtar, 2009, p. 14). Indeed, not only is there a paucity of scholarly toilet research, but there are many euphemistic names for the toilet, including hopper, Johnny, janey, loo, potty or privy, just as there are for defecation and urinating, e.g., taking a crap or dump, pooping, or doing a wee or draining the one-eyed monster. These euphemisms for "shitting and pissing" as many ordinary persons often call it (or the equivalent variants) suggest that the psychology of the toilet is not something that scholars and others want to straightforwardly speak about let alone investigate in depth (e.g., doctors refer to stools, feces or a bowel). Perhaps in part, this is because such topics are on the margins of the body that evoke both power and danger[3] within elaborate and complex cosmologies (e.g., moral values, social rules and metaphysical subjects) which excrement and urine symbolize, and thus a whole per- sonal domain of life becomes unspeakable, even unthinkable, as the celebrated anthropologist Mary Douglas noted (1966).

Thus, this book probes the private intimacies and prohibitions of private (and public) bathrooms (the latter is an example of the private in the public domain)[4], as well as the fantasies, meanings and scripts (to be deciphered), and use of what is euphemistically called excretion in other psychopathological and normative contexts. A number of clinical examples mainly taken from my psychoanalytic practice will expand and deepen my study. Indeed, in psychoanalytic theory and technique, defecation and urination have a wide range of "weird and wonderful" and all too human meanings that deserve additional ana- lytic exploration on their own terms, for they reveal, or at least sug- gest, everyday aspects of the human condition[5] that have largely been underappreciated if not ignored by analysts and others. Lacan, for instance, says that humans are the only animals that contemplate what to do with their excrement and urine after they finish their business. Such considerations significantly impact how analysands and others live their everyday existence, as well their efforts to fashion a flourishing life. For example, including toilet flushes that use water, the average human generates 4,000 gallons of urine a year and about 77 pounds of excrement without water; they also spend about three years of their life going to the toilet (George, 2008, pp. 19, 6).[6] The fact is, to some extent what makes us feel human, is our capacity to control our bodies in our ordinary lives, and using the toilet (or exploiting feces and urine in other contexts such as in sexual deviations say in the bedroom, or in public excretion such as open defecation in India or legally defined disorderly conduct in the U.S.), is one of the great instantiating moments of this autonomous capacity. From a societal perspective it has been claimed that how society deals with feces and urine ("waste management") is an index of its civility (e.g., how and what it defines as appropriate norms and socially deviant) (Weinberg & Williams, 2005). Indeed, the great American historian, sociologist and philosopher of technology, especially noted for his study of cities and urban architecture, Lewis Mumford wrote, "You can judge the quality of a civilization by the way it disposes of its waste" (Greed, 2010, p. 117). For example, as Slovenian Marxist-Lacanian philosopher Slavoj Žižek noted, there are important differences in the way that Germans, French and Anglo-Americans relate to excrement as evidenced by the architecture of their toilets (an art form of a sort that straightforwardly encounters the human body):

> In a traditional German toilet, the hole into which shit disappears after we flush is right at the front, so that shit is first laid out for us to sniff and inspect for traces of illness [almost everyone in western society looks at their feces before flushing, seemingly inspecting their "creation"].[7] In the typical French toilet, on the contrary, the hole is at the back, i.e. shit is supposed to disappear as quickly as possible. Finally, the American (Anglo-Saxon) toilet presents a synthesis, a mediation between these opposites: the toilet basin is full of water, so that the shit floats in it, visible, but not to be inspected. [...].
>
> (Žižek, 2008, p. 3)

Žižek opines that each of the aforementioned toilets is composed of a particular ideological-animated perception of how the person should relate to his fecal matter. Drawing from Hegel, Žižek says that the toilet experience reflects three divergent existential orientations: the reflective thoroughness of the Germans suggesting German conservatism; the revolutionary hastiness of the French, suggesting

French revolutionary radicalism; and the utilitarian pragmatism of the English (and Americans). Thus, in the most intimate realm of the person, we have "an ambiguous contemplative fascination [Germans]; a wish to get rid of it as fast as possible [French]; a pragmatic decision to treat it as ordinary and dispose of it in an appropriate way" [English] (ibid). In short, as the famous saying goes, the personal is political whether in the private or public bathroom (as Lacan noted, there is a politics of peeing, "Public life [is] subject [to] laws of urinary segregation") (Lacan, 1977, p. 151).

The bathroom or restroom as it is sometimes called becomes a tool for discerning how a society functions, that is, what it values, how it separates people from one another (e.g., man vs. woman; heterosexual vs. homosexual; transgender, transsexual and gender queer; and in the past, blacks and whites). In other words, how a society gets rid of its feces and urine, its sewage, conveys a lot about our politics, economics and religion. As Žižek notes elsewhere, quoting Erica Jong, "German toilets are really the key to the horrors of the Third Reich. People who can build toilets like this are capable of anything" (Jong, 1973, p. 35). Another example, the toilet euphemistically called the "throne" is believed to have emanated from King Louis XIV, who frequently attended to royal business while sitting on his toilet, regarding it as an acceptable substitute to his usual throne.[8] Today, the *Royal Toilet Throne* costs $11,977 and has been described by the sellers as:

> Reign supreme on the porcelain throne with this beautifully crafted royal toilet that is fit for a king. With medieval luxury, this wooden royal toilet throne includes a candle holder, ash tray, and even plays a musical chime as the toilet seat gloriously rises.
> (www.thisiswhyimbroke.com, royal-toilet-throne retrieved 11/12/20)

Needless to say, the customer who finds such a toilet appealing probably has some belief or fantasy (or childhood memory and affect) that makes such a purchase appear reasonable if not summoning to him.[9]

In this book, the first of its kind, I take up the psychology of the toilet in contemporary western society mainly from a contemporary psychoanalytic point of view, but frequently informed by sociological (and less so anthropological and architectural) insights, and empirical psychological findings. My main focus is on the ordinary person's everyday experience of defecating and urinating in the private and public bathroom, and other related atypical private and public contexts (e.g., as in sexual deviations, the so-called "perversions").

Drawing from the phenomenological tradition, our thoughts, emotions and behavior are always formed (if not greatly influenced), by the socio-historical context in which the person is actively involved (they reside in a situated existence steeped in a complicated social reality). In other words, phenomena, such as toileting, present themselves in a context-dependent and setting-specific manner, and it is the lived experience of the person, how they perceive things, makes them intelligible and responds to them that matters most (Aho, 2008). This includes, at least where it is possible to reasonably discern the personal fantasies, meanings and scripts (i.e., characters understood from behaving from described reasons) conscious and unconscious that motivate or at least in part, animate behavior and transform perception (Stoller, 1985, pp. 120, 119). I should note that my focus is on the toilet in the bathroom, not the sink, shower, bath or general décor, for these aspects of the bathroom deserve their special study (though of course, as part of the totality of circumstances of the toilet experience they have some bearing and will occasionally merit comment).[10]

The psychology of excretion has been touched upon in psychoanalysis in various clinical publications (but never as its own subject per se, let alone at book length), the anal phase and anal character (roughly referred to these days as Obsessive Compulsive Disorder ("OCD")), and toilet training being the most famous examples. However, in addition to exploring defecating and urinating in their diverse everyday contexts (normative and atypical), I also want to explore the seemingly far-fetched (at least to some) ideas of intimacy, cleanliness and pleasure that can render a toilet into something akin to a "sacred site," a place of everyday transcendence. For example, you regularly walk into a bathroom/toilet "unclean" (e.g., dirty bodies with a full bladder and bowel), and come out "clean" (e.g., cleanliness connected to bodily release/emptying of excess), a secular symbolic enactment of impurity and purity rituals, the latter leading to, or at least intrapsychically evoking a sense of integrity, unity and purity, as Douglas brilliantly pointed out (Douglas, 1966).[11]

Indeed, issues around aesthetics, hygiene and etiquette are at play in toilet behavior, sometimes embarrassingly so, but also sometimes as spiritually evocative and enhancing moments. As the great Chinese Taoist philosopher, on par with Lao Tzu, noted, "There is no place" the Way (the *Tao*, the One, that is natural, spontaneous, eternal, unnamable and ineffable) "doesn't exist... It is the piss and shit!" (perhaps this is shit and piss as a symbol of creative formlessness) (Watson, 1968, pp. 240–241). In other words, as with dirt, piss and shit have no universal and absolute singular meaning, let alone a negative one in a specific culture, it allows the possibility that defecating and urinating can be experienced as more than a mere necessary biological function that is satisfying (which is not to be underappreciated especially if you have trouble defecating or urinating).

In fact, more recently, the late Marco Frascari, a former professor of architecture at the University of Pennsylvania claimed that the purpose of architecture, especially that of bathrooms, including the toilet, "is to design a place of 'happiness'," that is, "a *vita beata*... a way of life free from impairment caused by psychic activity" (e.g., anxiety and stress such as shame, embarrassment, disgust). Frascari refers to such bathrooms as "numinous rooms where a *vita beata*, a 'happy' life can take place" (i.e., where relaxing, congenial and satisfying psychic activity can occur), the opposite of the typical institutional bathroom (especially public facilities, but also some apartments and homes) that is a "closet of secret constraints" (i.e., controlled, monitored and watched by infrared eyes, such as standardized automated, gazing flushometers, the speedy cleaning faucets and hand driers) and worse, that in no way evokes "transcendence," the "ethereal" and the "sacred" (Frascari, 1997, pp. 164, 166). In fact, these standardized/automated elements make personal doings feel very impersonal. What Frascari is arguing for, and I agree with him, is that the bathroom, specifically the toilet, can be viewed as a "holy dwelling" one that is not necessarily the case in the moral and rational sense, but rather "a non-rational place of well-being" that can be "therapeutic" on the way to a "beatific life" (ibid., p. 167). This notion of the toilet, of defecation and urination as being a potentially spiritual moment, has been memorialized for example, in Judaism's prayer "Ashar yatzar" ("who has formed man," read "all humans"). The function of the blessing is to thank God for having the natural capacity to defecate and urinate, for if not, life would not be possible to sustain. Other religions have similar kinds of gratitude-oriented prayers, emphasizing that even in the toilet there is the possibility of becoming spiritual elevated, if only briefly. It is also worth noting a rather extreme fact, that Martin Luther "reportedly ate a spoonful of his own excrement daily and wrote that he couldn't understand the generosity of a God who freely gave such important and useful remedies" to distressing skin ailments and the like (George, 2008, p. 8).[12] I am not advocating Luther's behavior, only pointing to the historical, perhaps psycho-spiritual link that some believe exists between excrement, health and God perceived as a Healer.[13]

Notwithstanding Frascari's rhetorical flourish—and who can see the overflowing toilet as angelic or the *Tao*—the fact is, he is making an important point that I believe is greatly underappreciated by analysts, and for that matter most people striving for a flourishing life, namely, that with the proper attunement to the totality of circumstances of the toileting experience, it can in certain instances be a place where "spirit is a living presence" (Frascari, 1997, p. 168). Indeed, in our day the "odor of sanctity" is unconsciously suggested when we use air fresheners, such as the fragrance of roses and incense, to make the toilet call to mind a numinous place (ibid). As I hope to suggest in this book, what is needed is the cultivation of the faculty of perception and intellectual intuition, somewhat similar to how one understands the dream. This is not so much fantasy-construction, but imaginative attunement to the symbols of the numinosity of the bathroom/toilet. Suggesting, where reasonable and plausible, how such imaginative perception and imaginative knowledge can become an imaginative consciousness in the bathroom/toilet (ibid., p. 180), is one of the unique features of this book.

While there have been many psychoanalytically oriented publications written about sex, eating, drinking and the like, there is no single volume that studies the toilet—the psychology of defecating and urinating in ordinary life, that is, in the everyday personal and social context, as well as in the clinical setting, and on its own terms. With regard to the latter for example, in my 36 years in psychoanalytic practice, I have had one patient write on my bathroom wall, "Marcus is the biggest asshole, a shit head" (presumably insulting my intelligence); a second patient left a huge bowel movement in the toilet which could not be flushed and I had to plunger it; another patient left her blood drenched tampon in the toilet; while another one masturbated into the toilet leaving traces of his dripping semen on the seat. There have been a few other examples of such behavior over the years but these come to mind. Incidentally, as I recollect, none of these patients was borderline, psychotic or even seriously delinquent teenagers. Many other patients refused to use the air spray, instead choosing to leave a stinky bathroom whose smell infected the waiting room. Obviously, the aforementioned examples were meant to convey a message to me and to my other patients (to state the obvious, a hostile one),[14] but such behavior was much more complicated in its depth and meanings when it was analytically explored.

Structure of the Book

Chapter Two, On Constipation, Diarrhea and Irritable Bowel Syndrome, provides three clinical vignettes that depict what having these conditions feels like. While all of these conditions are often mixed together, for heuristic purposes I have divided them so that the reader can get a sense of the unique ordeal of suffering the person goes through. Constipation is defined as when an individual has less than three bowel movements a week, or has difficult bowel movements. Diarrhea is defined as loose, watery stools that occur more often than usual. And Irritable Bowel Syndrome (IBS) is defined as an intestinal disorder causing pain in the belly, gas, diarrhea and constipation.

Chapter Three, Adult Female Urinary Incontinence, focuses on the suffering, the sense of humiliation and stigma, the impoverished self-concept and diminished self-esteem that is so common among women suffering from this condition. In particular, I discuss the social and recreational withdrawing from everyday life, worry and anxiety related to being incontinent in the public domain, depression, and diminished intimacy and physical/sexual proximity, that is so typical of adult female urinary incontinence. Some practical suggestions for improving how one better lives with the condition are provided.

Chapter Four, Toilet Cursing, focuses on the so-called "anal-phase" related cursing for that is the form that most cursing tends to take. Scatological means relating to or characterized by an attentiveness in excrement and excretion such as in scatological humor. Scatological language is regarded as a universal phenomenon, though what constitutes scatological in a particular culture is context-dependent and setting-specific. The symbolism of "shit" is discussed leading to the conclusion that while toilet cursing can be ill-conceived, ill-advised and ill-fated, it can also have a positive consequence for the person who curses and the listener (e.g., as part of the "carnivalesque"). Telephone scatologia, caprolalia (involuntary and repetitive use of obscene language as in Tourette's syndrome), and caprophagia (eating excrement) are also discussed from a clinical point of view.

Chapter Five, Public Bathroom Graffiti, discusses graffiti as being a kind of "living Rorschach", depicting what the author feels and thinks, in a few lines or perhaps an accompanying picture. I further discuss why people do graffiti and its consequence for the anonymous author and anonymous reader. Scatological graffiti, like all types of bathroom graffiti, can usefully be conceptualized as derivatives from the repressed, similar to dreams, jokes and slips of the tongue. That is, such graffiti whether viewed as storytelling, artistic expression or play, seems to centrally express anally-based and animated sexual and aggressive material.

In Chapter Six, Toilet Humor, I focus on the subject of toilet, potty or scatological humor, and suggest that there is more to this form of humor than is usually realized by the average person. I provide a word on the developmental aspects of toilet humor, that is, the role of such humor in children through adolescence and beyond. Next, I provide a hypothesis on why such humor is funny to the adult, and why some adults can't appreciate such humor and might be better off if they could. Finally, I suggest that toilet humor has something to teach us about the human condition, about our collective anxieties and fears, and the possibility of the "transcendentally human."

Chapter Seven, The Personal Meaning of Urinating and Defecation, attempts to convey the deeply personal nature of urinating and defecating as seen in men who have an enlarged prostate, prisoner's being subjected to "excremental assault" in the Nazi concentration camps, and in the dreams of three of my patients. In all of these contexts, we see how urine and excrement are hugely psychologically freighted for better or worse.

Notes

1 Incidentally, Hitler, Napoleon and Chairman Mao also had rectal difficulties so serious they sometimes interrupted their murderous careers (Blumer, 2013, p. 9).
2 Anthropological evidence indicates that ancient Greeks and Romans willingly defecated communally and used their left hand to wipe, mainly for superstitious reasons.
3 Though in some instances the same excreta can be viewed as funny.
4 While using public toilets is a private matter, it should never be forgotten that this private behavior has wide ranging public ripples in terms of hygiene, sanitation and the like. Currently, there is no "systems theory about sanitation" that could solve this world problem (George, 2008, p. 237). It is worth mentioning the "fears" associated with using public bathrooms, especially during a global pandemic, are reality-based.
5 What constitutes "the human condition" is of course perspectival and must be understood within the context of the episteme, the socio-intellectual reality of the era one is referencing. Strictly speaking, there is no human condition, except in a specific socio-historical context.
6 Worth noting, by 2050, half of the planet's estimated 8.9 billion people will live in nations that are chronically short of water, let alone drinkable water (George, 2008, p. 227).
7 It is worth mentioning that some have claimed that verbal abuse connected to the anal zone is particularly accentuated in Germany (and the U.S.). In the German context, this is probably because such abuse expresses a cultural value assigned to cleanliness (Haslam, 2012).
8 In the White House President Lyndon Johnson carried on the tradition, in line with his approach to leadership. He once told a prospective applicant for a job as his assistant: "I don't want loyalty, I want LOYALTY. I want you to kiss my ass in Macy's window at high noon and tell me it smells like roses." In other words, the toilet was used as a very public seat of power (Blumer, 2013, p. 62).

9 Incidentally, the most expensive toilet on record was the toilet designed by NASA's space shuttles which cost $23.4 million dollars (George, 2008, p. 225).

10 The contemporary bathroom with a tub, sink and a toilet is a fairly recent innovation. It wasn't until about mid 1950s that most homes in the U.S. had such a designated room.

11 An interesting question is how clean is clean? That is, how are these distinctions reasonably made?

12 Likewise, in earlier times of Tibetan Buddhism, the excrement of the Dalai Lama, Tibet's living God, was viewed as having magical healing powers. His holy excrement was dried and put in amulets, sometimes used as medicine and even as a condiment to be sprinkled on food (Blumer, 2013, p. 21).

13 It should be noted that in Erikson's study of Luther, Erikson indicated that Luther complained of frequent constipation much of his life as well as urinary retention problems, though he had his main spiritual revelations about faith and the like while sitting on the toilet (Erikson, 1958). From the sublime to the tragic, the great Elvis Presley died on the toilet of a heart attack.

14 In Jung's memoir, he reports that as a young student he felt horror while obsessively gazing at a cathedral that he wanted to stop looking at because he was anxious he would commit a terrible desecration. Three days went by, and after making numerous attempts to deflect his obsessively sinful thoughts he gave in, he imagined God seated on his royal gold throne, letting go of a huge "turd" smack onto the cathedral (1963, as cited in Haslam, 2012). One wonders if Jung had some kind of Oedipal issue at play, the "puny" Jung and the omnipotent God.

References

Aho, K. (2008). Medicalizing Mental Health. A Phenomenological Alternative. *Journal of Medical Humanity* 29, 243–259.

Akhtar, S. (2009). *Comprehensive Dictionary of Psychoanalysis*. London: Karnac.

Blumer, R.H. (2013). *Wiped. The Curious History of Toilet Paper*. New York: Middlemarch Media Press.

Douglas, M. (1966). *Purity and Danger*. London: Routledge.

Eigen, M. (2022). Festering: Mini-moments, *Psychoanalytic Review*, 109 (2), June, 91–96.

Erikson, E.H. (1958). *Young man Luther: a study in psychoanalysis and history*, London: Faber.

Frascari, M. (1997). The Pneumatic Bathroom. In N. Lahiji and D.S. Friedman (eds) *Plumbing. Sounding modern architecture*. New York: Princeton Architectural Press, 162–180.

Freud, S. (1913). Foreword. In J.G. Bourke and L.P. Kaplan (eds) *The Portable Scatolog. Excerpts from Scatological Rites of All Nations* [1891]. New York: William Morrow and Company, Inc, 1994, 5–9.

George, R. (2008). *The Big Necessity. The Unmentionable World of Human Waste and Why It Matters*. New York: Henry Hold and Company.

Greed, C. (2010). Creating a Nonsexist Restroom. In H. Molotch and L. Noren (eds) *Toilet. Public Restrooms and the Politics of Sharing*, New York: New York University Press, 239–252.

Haslam, N. (2012). *Psychology in the Bathroom*. New York: Palgrave Macmillan.

Jones, E. (1961). *The Life and Work of Sigmund Freud*. Edited and abridged in one volume by L. Trilling and S. Marcus. Volume 1, New York: Basic Books.

Jong, E. (1973). *Fear of Flying. A Novel*. New York: Henry Holt & Company.

Jung, C.J. (1963). *Memoirs, dreams, reflections* (rev. edn.) New York: Pantheon.

Kaplan, R.M. (2010). Freud's excellent adventure Down Under: The only publication in Australia by the founder of psychoanalysis. *Australasian Psychiatry*, 18, 205–209.

Lacan, J. (1977) *Ecrits: A Selection*, trans. A. Sheridan. New York: Norton.

Molotch, H. (2010). Introduction. In H. Molotch and L. Noren (eds) *Toilet. Public Restrooms and the Politics of Sharing*, New York: New York University Press, 1–20.

Penner, B. (2010). Entangled with a User. Inside Bathrooms with Alexander Kira and Peter Greenway. In H. Molotch and L. Noren (eds) *Toilet. Public Restrooms and the Politics of Sharing*, New York: New York University Press, 239–252.

Stoller, R. (1985). *Observing the Erotic Imagination*. New Haven, CT: Yale University Press.

Watson, B., trans. (1968). *The Complete Works of Chuang Tzu*. New York: Columbia University Press.

Weinberg, M.S. & Williams, C.J. (2005). Fecal matters: Habitus, embodiments and deviance. *Social Problems*, 52, 315–336.

Žižek, S. (2008). *The Plague of Fantasies*. London: Verso.

Chapter 2

On Constipation, Diarrhea and Irritable Bowel Syndrome

In this chapter, rather than review the mainly psychological literature on the aforementioned conditions, which is readily available,[1] I will present three case vignettes, one on constipation, the other on diarrhea and the final one on Irritable Bowel Syndrome (aka IBS). In IBS symptoms include abdominal pain, bloating, constipation and diarrhea. Though some people can regulate their symptoms by managing diet, lifestyle and stress, others will require prescription and over the counter medication. Psychotherapy is also sometimes sought to get some relief. The causes of IBS are hardly known however, there are about 200,000 cases diagnosed each year in the U.S. For the most part, the diagnosis is made by symptoms. IBS can either be more of the constipation or diarrhea type, or a mixture of the two. Whether one has chronic constipation, diarrhea or IBS, it is accurate to say that the patient is going through an ordeal of daily suffering.

Vignette 1: Constipation

John was a 45-year-old Caucasian, Catholic man referred by his gastro intestinal (GI) doctor who had become frustrated with John because his constipation came and went and he never settled down for long periods of time constipation free. This meant many visits to the GI doctor and a patient who was frequently in distress. John, a professor was married to a part-time lawyer and they had three children, age 15, 11 and 9 who appeared to be doing well in school and home and were generally high functioning. The children did complain that "Daddy was not around enough." John came to me because of his constipation but also because he had gone through a number of significant losses in his life, his best friend died from Covid-19 while his beloved cat also died a few months later. He also lost two other friends from his list of casual friends. John claimed that he felt bereft

DOI: 10.4324/9781003219705-2

by these losses. He was also having problems at work, where he felt his colleagues were jealous of his success as a published writer, often not knowing how to deal with their anger at him and their efforts to "jam" him up in terms of the politics of the department. John's marriage was satisfactory, though he noted that his wife was getting tired of his endless complaining about being constipated, spending inordinate amounts of time in the bathroom "trying to make" as he told me. John said his wife was not as demonstrative towards him or the children as he would like a bit more affection like a hug or kiss when he came home from work. John was seen three times a week in psychoanalysis for about three years and the treatment was a partial success because his constipation lessened by the time the treatment was completed. In addition, his self-esteem and self-concept improved as his anxiety and depression was lessened. John came from a family of professionals, he had a good relationship with his parents and his two older siblings who lived near-bye and had children.

The treatment began with John telling me that he thought that his GI doctor was sick of him due to his repeated visits that usually involved new medicines that worked for a while but were fundamentally unhelpful. John did not need much convincing from me that his constipation was influenced by his psychology but he was clueless as to how. His GI doctor told me that if I could keep John away from him, except when really necessary, he would be appreciative. John also said that he was prone to depression, and he began the third session with a dream:

> I dreamt that I was in a "field of dreams" having a baseball catch with my father who was criticizing me how I threw the ball. I tried to perfect my throwing the ball back to him, but was not able to. My father got angry at me for being so feeble but I told him I was trying my best. I then began to feel like I had to go to the toilet, in fact the pooh was about to go into my under wear. I stopped everything, ran into the house to get to the toilet but nothing came out. I woke up in a near panic that I would not be able to go to the toilet and would have to endure this situation forever. The thought of being this clogged up was "horrifying" to me.

John's main association to the dream was that his father appeared to him as being too harsh on him and not being willing and able to give him a compliment about his throwing the ball. He said that his father could be critical, controlling and altogether a perfectionist (his father worked on Wall Street). After discussing the dream John indicated that he could not feel much affection for his father and actually did not want to have a catch with him anymore. He claimed that it was as if his father was constipated in terms of not being able to let go of his defensive regime and compliment, or at least be supportive of his son when he was clearly trying his best. When I asked John what came to mind about the constipation in the dream he told me, that he felt as if he were manifesting a symptom that actually belonged to his father who was so unforthcoming He also associated to the fact that he could be more of a withholder than his father when it came to constipation.

As the treatment unfolded John's anger at his father for being emotionally withholding began to bother him more. John also indicated however, that he was afraid of his father as a child, for he was a tall man and very demanding in terms of getting good grades and doing well in after school activities like sports. In fact, I offered the interpretation to John that perhaps him being more constipated than his father, as implied in the dream, was an Oedipal victory of a sort. That is, the fact that John was more often constipated than his father meant that he was better than his father in at least something. In the transference, John would often experience me as overbearing, as talking too much and as emotionally distant, similar to how he experienced his father and to a lesser extent his wife.

In a later session, the Oedipal theme came up again, and it was connected to his constipation from time to time. For example, John began to realize that his holding on to his pooh was a way of keeping himself whole and safe from his father, wife and for that matter everyone else. In other words, to "let go" of his feces was roughly equivalent to him being broken inside. This also linked up with the panic in the dream when he thought that he would be constipated forever, an unconscious reference I thought to this being his only way of avoiding castration. John also wondered if his irritation at his competitive university colleagues who were inclined to ignore or put down his writing output was connected to this in that he felt that they were castrating in their way of being with him. It wasn't clear what he did with this anger, probably it was turned inwards, one of his common defenses (e.g., his depression and holding in the feces).

John also came to realize that his withholding his feces was a way of not giving, and not giving into his childhood parents (and current father and mother), and in his current life mainly his wife, and to a lesser extent his children who complained that he was not around enough. That is, John felt he was giving much more than he was getting at home with his wife and children and at the university with his jealous and competitive colleagues. By withholding his feces John was in effect protesting his lack of getting by not giving up his pooh, which would have delighted his wife, parents who were aware of his chronic constipation and even the GI doctor.

John's constipation went through an ordeal of suffering when he was so backed up he got an impacted bowel requiring digital manipulation by the GI doctor followed by two fleet enemas to clear out his bowel which was causing him excruciating pain. John's wife gave him the enemas and he noted that he had cleverly unconsciously manipulated her to be a giver to him. It took a few days until John made a proper bowel movement but only after having to wear an adult diaper due to the seepage from the enema and his constipation. Wearing this diaper was chastening to John who experienced the diaper as a humiliation, especially to his wife and his parents who found this out when he told them about it. When I asked him why he would tell this to his mother and father he acknowledged that it was "dumb," a way of inflicting self-castration for his father (and mother) to see. In the transference John experienced me at this time as a benign figure who wanted the best for him, though he sometimes slipped into viewing me as the castrating father such as when I asked him couldn't he have found an alternative solution to the adult diaper if it bothered him so much.

Another theme related to his constipation, was his loss of his friend and cat all within the Covid-19 pandemic. John acknowledged that he felt he had lost an important part of his world of meaning when his best friend suddenly died. This death, and his beloved cat's death, all within the context of the pandemic, which meant the loss of normal life as John knew it, contributed to his sense of incomplete mourning and depression. Retaining his bowel movement thus appeared to be an unconscious way to "hold on" to what he lost. John felt this interpretation was plausible as he told me and it set him thinking of the connection between loss and constipation.

By the third year of treatment John became more willing and able to get his wife to be more demonstrative to him, as well as his parents. Correlated with these developments was the fact that he was less depressed and therefore, was less in need of turning his aggression on himself in terms of the distressing aspects of his constipation. This led to John beginning to become more regular in the frequency of his bowel movements. Not only that, but this development seemed to be correlated with John becoming more of a giver to his wife and while at the same time making more time to be with his kids who previously complained about his emotional remoteness and practical absence in their lives.

As the treatment progressed John revealed some embarrassing information as he described it, the fact that he would watch pornography while masturbating including anal or rectal digging. John said that he liked the sensation of putting his finger up his anus while masturbating giving him a sense of extreme pleasure. At the same time, John told me that he was inclined to anal intercourse with his wife, who while she did not like it, participated in it. John's masturbation and anal/rectal digging were related to an early experience he had while in camp where a counselor molested him by "dick assing" him as he called it, which he found terrifying and pleasurable at the same time. Thus, the masturbation was a partial repetition of his traumatic experience, though he was now the active participant not the passive victim. Likewise, we viewed his penchant for anal intercourse as a reaction formation in that it was he who unconsciously wanted to be anally penetrated by his father. That is, John had the fantasy of being sodomized by his father while on the "field of dreams." The fact that he reversed the main thrust of the anal intercourse, from passive to active supported this hypothesis. It also helped account for why he also wanted his wife to put her finger up his anus while he masturbated though it did not come to ejaculation.

As the treatment progressed, and John's depression and constipation lessened his penchant for masturbation, pornography and anal intercourse lessened. He also felt less guilty for his provocative fantasies. In the transference, I sometimes became the brute of a father who wanted to dominate him into submission.

While John ended treatment after three years, his constipation did lessen in frequency and intensity. He also took greater responsibility for his symptoms by changing what he could in his lifestyle, stress level, exercise and diet. While of course he was aware that these factors may have played a role in his condition, he always relied on the GI doctor to guide him, almost as if he was a child relating to a caring parent. By John using simple stool softeners, eating more fiber, exercising more often and learning how to meditate when he was in a panic or near panic, he was able to reduce the frequency and intensity of his constipation and increase his feeling of well-being.

Vignette Two: Diarrhea

Janet, age 28, a Caucasian Jewish woman, lived in Brooklyn with her boyfriend who worked in a "start-up." She worked in public relations and found her job to be hard going, in part due to her "crazy" boss who intimidated her as she described him. She could not leave her job mainly for financial reasons. Janet was self-referred through a recommendation from a friend and was in treatment three times a week for about two years. Her main complaint was that she had "free-floating" anxiety, headaches, tiredness and on and off again diarrhea, a symptom that she was most distressed about because it interfered with her functioning at work and in her personal life.

At work Janet was frequently "running" to the bathroom and felt an abiding sense of anxiety that she would lose control of her feces and soil herself, which did happen from time to time. She thus always brought a change of underwear to work and cleaning wipes to be prepared for the worst. Janet said that her diarrhea was worst at work when her boss would criticize her and raised his voice. At these moments she felt anger at usually being unfairly targeted and fear of losing her job. When I suggested to her that her anger may manifest itself in her body, that is, in her diarrhea, she agreed. She and I came to the hypothesis that at these moments her diarrhea represented her wish to symbolically get rid of her boss through her diarrhea. "Getting rid of him in a big mess down the toilet" as I noted.

This being said, Janet felt out of control of her body, and her anger felt similarly. Janet had difficulty expressing her anger in assertive behavior and she believed that one of the reasons she was targeted by her boss as his scapegoat was that she appeared like an easy target, that is, she had low self-esteem, was dependent-like and had significant difficulties standing up for herself (though she could be a creative marketer). She also felt "shitty" about herself not only because her boss made her feel that way but because she was angry and upset at her own helplessness, and "brokenness" at her inability to assert herself. She felt like a mess inside, symbolically expressed in the symptom.

Janet described her parents as adequate though she has numerous run-ins with her father who was overbearing and controlling. Her father worked in banking she said, and he was used to being in charge of many employees, hence, he could be dictatorial with Janet and her older brother. Her brother was married with children and worked in banking also, and had a tenuous relationship with her father. Janet said that her mother was fairly nurturing and stable, though under her father's control, which often bothered her and her brother because she would not stand up for Janet when her father was picking on her as she viewed it.

Janet's diarrhea began after a botched colon-rectal surgery that she had when she was about age 9. As a result of the surgery, she spent much of her childhood with diarrhea due to a lack of complete control of her bowel function. She told me about one instance, when she was about age 10, that while walking home from school she felt she had to go to the toilet, but as she was too far from home to defecate, she went in a trash can of a neighbor's house that had an open garage. Janet described, in riveting language, how anxious she felt that she would be caught by the anonymous neighbor doing her "business." Janet said that this kind of thing (having nowhere to do her business) happened more often than she wanted to remember and it was only when she became a young adult that her bowel control became somewhat normalized. Janet described the aforementioned episodes as humiliating, and she often wondered how she functioned in school (she was "ok" academically) where she felt chronically distracted by her anxiety that she would lose control and soil herself. Overall, from an early age Janet had feelings of being out of control, and broken in some kind of way. Moreover, she had a fear of being "caught" in her "shittiness," for example, by peers at school and later at work, if they might be able to smell something. This shame contributed to her feelings of being bad and messed up inside and magnified the wish not to reveal herself and her true feelings.

Another manifestation of Janet's diarrhea was her tendency to get rid of things that she had no use for, sometimes this sounded rather over-the-top to me. For example, once when Janet was re-arranging her studio apartment because she felt it was too messy and the like, she took a perfectly adequate lamp that she could not find a place for, and threw it into the garbage. "Out of sight, out of mind" she told me. When I pointed out that what she did seemed rather extreme, she agreed, but the feeling of being out of control of her apartment's décor was stronger than any other consideration so she got rid of the lamp without any ambivalence. I pointed out to Janet that she had trouble "keeping things in," especially "good" things, somewhat like her diarrhea. She more or less agreed with my interpretation and added that she had difficulty in holding on to positive feelings about herself as it was as if they turned bad inside her.

About her personal life, Janet noted that she had a hard time keeping relationships going, having had many boyfriends but for one reason or another, she found fault with all of them, at least until she found her current live-in boyfriend of one year. This being said, Janet indicated that she wanted to break up with her boyfriend, saying that he was not nurturing and stable enough for a woman like herself who needed a lot of demonstrativeness that he loved her. She claimed that her boyfriend was inhibited and remote too often. Janet admitted that she had difficulties in giving and receiving love, and often wanted to end relationships because she felt claustrophobic. When I pointed out to Janet that she seemed to have had a tendency to get rid of things and people sooner than later, similar to her diarrhea symptom, she tended to agree, though she felt powerless to do anything about it. That is, her anxiety grew and grew, so she felt she had to act accordingly, frequently feeling guilty for prematurely ending her close relationships with significant others. In the transference, her wish to get rid of me as a psychotherapist, was something that she often threatened, finding our regular meetings three times a week as too intense, and thus she felt claustrophobic. Again, it was only when I pointed out to her not only the fear of being controlled by the malignant boss, but also the possible link to her diarrhea, that she made the connection between her feeling that there was "shit inside" her that needed to be expelled, and her difficulty internalizing me as a "good object," and that she wanted to expel me similar to her diarrhea, that she settled down into the therapy.

Janet also wanted to be given to by her significant others, and most other people too, but she had great difficulty holding on to it, that is, she had a tendency to turn what was given into shit which she can't hold onto, but who wants to hold onto shit anyway? In other words, Janet felt shitty but externalizes this feeling, and then believes everybody is shitty not giving her anything good.

However, it was in the realm of her sexual life that Janet's diarrhea, and anxiety about her diarrhea became an interfering factor. Janet told me that she had great difficulty having sexual relations with her boyfriend, and other men before that, because she was afraid of losing control and soiling herself. For this and other reasons, Janet had great difficulty having an orgasm, and letting her boyfriend do cunnilingus to her. Her anxiety about losing control at these moments was too intense for her to relax into a man pleasuring her. When I asked her how she felt about the aforementioned she noted that she felt lonely and alone, even though she was the one who was implementing the inhibition. Janet then linked her fear of intimacy with her diarrhea symptom, in that in both instances there was a fear of losing bodily control. Not only did she lose control of her sexuality but she also lost control of her aggression, at least in fantasy.

Janet did describe one instance when she did soil herself a little bit during sexual intercourse. She indicated that while her boyfriend was mounting her in the missionary position, she farted and some liquid pooh came out of her, embarrassing her greatly. She ran to the bathroom and then cleaned up the small mess on the sheets. Janet said that her boyfriend did not make a "big deal" about the mishap though she was extremely embarrassed. Interestingly Janet said that her boyfriend was aware of her diarrhea symptom but learned to live with it, other boyfriends she had tried to conceal the symptom from. Janet and I viewed the aforementioned as a symbolic expression of her feelings of badness for her instinctual wishes and guilt and shame at them. We also understood her fear of being controlled by men by considering the possibility that the disorder was an expression of her declaring that she could not be controlled.

By the second year of treatment Janet's diarrhea began to lessen in frequency and intensity and more importantly perhaps, she felt that she could regulate her anxiety before she felt the urge to do her business. In other words, in part due to our discussions, Janet began to feel that she had some control over her body and over the sources of her anxiety, and therefore she felt she had more control over her destiny. Her behavior at work and with her boyfriend also seemed to improve, though I felt that she ended the treatment way too prematurely.

Vignette Three: Irritable Bowel Syndrome

Bill, age 40, a single, Caucasian Catholic man lived alone in Queens. He came to me via his GI doctor who indicated that Bill would come to see him countless times with diffuse complaints regarding his IBS, complaints that appeared to him to be real but exaggerated in his discomfort level. As a result, said the doctor, he was not able to do much to help Bill and he thought psychotherapy could be useful as an adjunct to the medications and diet he was on. I saw Bill for about two years, twice a week in supportive, psychoanalytically oriented psychotherapy. Bill was a cooperative patient in terms of coming to his sessions and paying his bill promptly. He said he had been suffering from anxiety and depression for years as well as IBS.

Bill worked as a compliance officer in a corporate setting, finding his job "ok" but "very stressful." As he told me, "getting other people to do what they are supposed to do is never easy," and he was usually the one who had to make sure work was done properly according to the rules. This meant that there were many colleagues who were often annoyed at him for pointing out their failures and mishaps, and his knit-picking in their view. Bill had high ambitions as a young man to be the head administrator at a large teaching hospital, but as his ambitions got frustrated he moved from job to job, feeling like a failure or at least an under functioning employee. Indeed, Bill impressed me as someone who was functioning below his capacity, middle management, as he was an extremely bright and capable person, though rather quirky and inhibited by his generalized anxiety. Bill had good reasons for feeling anxious and depressed. His mother was only sporadically nurturing and stable and her marriage to his father was in danger of divorce for as long as he could remember while growing up. The parents argued continually about this and that. Bill's mother would have rages at him for his minor infractions and punish him severely without listening to his side of events. His father usually stayed out of it, and did not protect Bill from his wife's raging and other obnoxious episodes. In part, as a result of the aforementioned Bill reported feeling generalized anxiety for as long as he could remember and depressed about the mediocrity of his life. He also had many obsessive and compulsive characteristics which impressed me as in play as a way of containing his anxiety and depression. For example, he was impeccably dressed, spoke in short clipped sentences and was fussy about details. Bill could also be obstinate, withholding and a minimizer from what I could tell. For example, his apartment had no pictures on the wall as he liked it that way because it was easy to clean the house he told me.

Bill reported that his first experience of IBS was probably when he was about age 7, when he was living with what sounded like his Borderline mother and accomplished scholar but passive father, and three brothers, in the affluent suburbs. His brothers sounded dysfunctional to me in different ways. Specifically, Bill reports that from about age 7 to 12, when he was being looked after by his babysitter, the woman would regularly expose her big breasts to him and he would put his face in between them. Bill indicated that this experience was both terrifying and pleasurable, especially when he was a near teenager. He acknowledged that he would frequently masturbate using the babysitter as his imagining. Bill says he never shared this information about the babysitter with his parents or anyone else and kept it a secret until he told me.

In part, as a result of the aforementioned traumatic experience, Bill said that he tended to avoid close relationships with women and men. In fact, the only major sexual experience he told me about in some detail was when he went to a prostitute in Las Vegas as a young adult. When he told me about this, he indicated that the prostitute did not charge him for her services, what turned out to be a lie as he later told me. Bill said he lied about the payment because he was embarrassed that he sunk so low as to go to a prostitute and didn't want me to think badly about him. When I pointed out that the lie was as significant in terms of his therapy as the deed itself, Bill acknowledged that he would regularly frequent prostitutes to get some relief from his loneliness. Bill did date women from time to time, even having sex with them, but he always regarded these women as just objects to be used to satisfy his physical needs. He never had a relationship with a significant other that lasted more than a few months.

With regards to his relationships with men, Bill had only one person he considered a friend, someone he spoke to a few times a year, an accountant, who sounded as dysfunctional as Bill was. While Bill was a likeable fellow, smart, witty, charming and self-satirizing, for the most part, he kept his distance from men. He told me that he usually declined going to lunch with colleagues and on the weekends, he spent most of the time doing errands and going to the movies alone.

Bill thus, impressed me as a loner type person. He thought himself ugly and fat, though I judged him as above average in looks and not at all seriously overweight. When I would point out the discrepancy between his self-concept and my perception of him, he would tell me that I was simply being kind to him: "What girl would want to date an ugly and fat man like myself," he would often tell me. As a result of this self-hatred, he would avoid relationships with women, even when he would fantasize about them in masturbatory and ordinary contexts, and attractive women were seeking him out, he usually declined their advances: "They must have pitied me," he told me, though I thought he was just being avoidant with them and evasive with me.

Bill said that he was both anxious and depressed that his personal life was so empty. He told me that "deep down" he wanted to have a girlfriend and then wife and children but was too afraid to get close to them or allow them to get too close to him. In fact, he told me about an unusual episode that when as a younger man he was engaged to a woman who he wanted to continue seeing but did not want to marry. Eventually, he gave in and agreed to marriage, except about a month into the engagement he developed a near impossible to believe symptom. He presented with a hysterical-like symptom of not being able to use his right arm properly. I interpreted this symptom as a form of castration anxiety, though the symptom, which did not have any physical causation, subsided after he called off the engagement.

I mention this episode because it indicates to what an extent Bill used his body to express his emotional state rather than verbalizing his concerns, this being a typical characteristic of many people suffering with IBS (and constipation or diarrhea). That is, the pathway from mind to body was permeable in the extreme. As Bill told me, whether he was stressed out about work or anxious and depressed about his impoverished personal life, his body would register the distress in some kind of bodily problem such as constipation or diarrhea. Bill further noted that he could not see a pattern to whether he would get constipation or diarrhea but he sensed either way, that it was his body's way of communicating his emotional distress. Bill hated his body, it felt like it was his enemy, making him feel unwell nearly every day with gas, constipation or diarrhea.

Bill indicated that his constipation bothered him a bit more than his proneness to diarrhea though he was chronically anxious that he would defecate on himself and/or not make it to the bathroom to do his business, both at work and when he was socially out. He always brought with him a change of under ware and a washcloth so he could clean himself up. Bill told me about how anxious he felt about his constipation, even once recently staying up the entire night on the toilet trying to go. During that time, he would engage in anal/rectal digging to loosen the stool and strained himself to get it to be released. Eventually, after going to the GI doctor who digitally manipulated him, and after a few enemas, he went to the toilet to relieve himself.

Bill impressed me as a rather neurotic type person. He was very "OCD'ish" in his way of comporting himself. He was always on time to the sessions, paid his bill on time and had his overall life at work and home very well organized. Too organized, hardly ever being spontaneous. Bill could not tolerate my being a few minutes late, even two or three minutes; on one occasion when I was late he put his check on my office desk and then harangued me for being late. When I asked him why he was so anxious and angry about my being two or three minutes late, he told me that being late showed a lack of respect for him and it reflected a disorganized therapist! I could not convince Bill that his anxious, angry demand was rather severe and that as we could make up the time at the end of the session the lateness should not be such a big deal to him. Nevertheless, after this one experience, I never was late again. We used this incident to explore the severity of his super-ego, his strictures against my lateness (however minimal), but also against himself and the inordinate demands he put on himself. We further explored this intense judgmentalism as connected to his severe and demanding mother where even minor lapses in behavior could elicit rage.

In treatment, Bill tended to view me as a benign but ineffective therapist because I was not able to correct his condition he said. That is, in the transference, I was regarded as similar to his father, smart but remote, and not up to snuff in dealing with his main IBS symptoms. Eventually he began to respect me when his symptoms lessened.

The treatment allowed Bill's symptoms to lessen by helping him focus on his generalized anxiety and assisting him to learn how to detect likely patterns to his constipation, diarrhea and bloating flare-ups. He came to understand that his anxiety was associated with his babysitter molesting him and his difficulty in managing the over-stimulation, the helplessness, rage and sexual arousal. He also gained greater understanding of the role his unpredictable mother played in the severity of his demands on himself and others. He became aware of how his constipation was correlated with his anger for example at his colleagues at work who were not doing their job adequately. The extent of his anger and his need to control it was manifested through his body, thus he had to control his anger so as not to "shit" all over his colleagues and hence ended up with constipation. The diarrhea tended to flare up when his anxiety was more prominent in areas where he felt he would be judged as being ineffective and damaged as the diarrhea made him feel. The treatment offered him a narrative of self-identity that he could use to mentally process his upset and conflicts rather than for them to be symbolically represented in uncomfortable bodily symptoms.

Final Comments

I have tried to give the reader a sense of the way of being-in-the-world that a patient who suffers from constipation, diarrhea and IBS tends to inhabit. It is a miserable existence. Given the scope of this book, I have focused on the psychological factors, the intra-psychic dynamics as they unfolded in a psychoanalytic psychotherapeutic context. In particular, I have stressed the importance of self-identity and the instinctual world of sex and aggression and the defenses against them. The overarching goal of treatment is to help the patient gain greater understanding of his internal world so he can develop a mental representation of what is going on and therefore, is less likely to bypass the mental and enact his conflict in the physical realm. This being said, I am well aware that any approach to patients suffering from the aforementioned conditions is best served by a wholistic approach. That is, a biopsychosocial framework (Muscatello, et. al., 2016). Indeed, my vignettes have been "narratively smoothed" a bit for the sake of clarity and intelligibility, but the fact is that most patients suffering from these distressing conditions have a range of psychological, developmental, biological, environmental and social factors at play in a complex interrelated, interdependent and interactive manner. They also often suffer from other conditions that makes treating them challenging (i.e., co-morbid conditions). What is clear is that the GI track is an incredibly fertile breeding ground for the development of later neurotic conflict, as well as other problems in living.

Note

1 See Haslam's fine review of the psychological literature in his interesting book (Haslam, 2012).

References

Haslam, N. (2012). *Psychology in the Bathroom.* New York: Palgrave Macmillan.
Muscatello, M.R.A., Bruno, A., Mento, C., Pandolfo, G., Zoccali, R.A. (2016). Personality traits and emotional patterns in irritable bowel syndrome. *World Journal of Gastroenterology*, 22 (28), 6402–6415.

Chapter 3

Adult Female Urinary Incontinence

Urinary incontinence in women is an all too common difficulty. As women get older, the prevalence and severity of its expression tends to increase (Debus & Kastneer, 2015, p. 165). For example, regarding nursing home residents, the frequency of urinary incontinence is roughly between 43% and 77%, 6% to 10% of all admissions. In addition, about 45% of all pregnant women become incontinent at some point in their pregnancy (ibid, p. 166). Urinary incontinence is thus a serious health difficulty in our ever-growing ageing society, and it is often not spoken about by the woman due to embarrassment and the like, to their health care provider, making the treatment that much more expensive as the situation worsens (ibid). The International Continence Society has defined incontinence as follows: "the complaint of any involuntary loss of urine" (Kuoch et al, 2019, p. 25).

In this chapter, I will be focusing on female incontinence in part, because it is "much more common in women than in men—among individuals younger than 65, nearly seven times as many women as men experience it" (Pettit & Chen, 2021, p. 94). By suffering I mean incontinence causes the woman to feel a sense of humiliation and stigma, diminished self-esteem and an impoverished self-concept, "social and recreational withdrawal, fear and anxiety related to being incontinent in public, depression or other psychological morbidity and reduced intimacy, affection and physical proximity" (Tranquility, 2016, n.p.). There are five types of incontinence: "urgency incontinence", which is the "sudden, compelling need to pass urine which is difficult to defer"; "overflow incontinence", which is "due to sudden increase in intra-abdominal or bladder (detrusor overactivity) pressure in over-distention of bladder"; "functional incontinence", which refers to "patients who have intact urinary storage functions, but are physically unable to reach [the] bathroom in time to pass urine (e.g., due to arthritis)"; "stress urinary incontinence", which is "urinary

DOI: 10.4324/9781003219705-3

incontinence during physical exertion (e.g., exercise) or due to coughing or sneezing" (the most common type in women); and finally, "mixed urinary incontinence," incontinence "that is associated with or preceded by urgency urinary incontinence, in addition to physical exertion, coughing or sneezing" (Kuoch et al., 2019, p. 26). Regardless of which type of incontinence one has, the personal and social impact on the person is usually powerful. Moreover, there is a range of medical treatments available (though incontinence is not technically a disease but a condition), but a lack of consensus about which treatment is best for one of the aforementioned five subtypes, adding further stress on the woman sufferer.

In this chapter I want to concentrate on the everyday "inner experience" of female incontinence, for regardless of the subtype, they all involve the same problem, "the complaint of any involuntary loss of urine" (Kuoch et al, 2019, p. 25). Moreover, the woman has to contend with dire consequences of incontinence for personal and social existence. I therefore will discuss female incontinence in general terms, though when I am specifically referring to one of the aforementioned subtypes I will identify it as such.

I will be organizing the material to be presented in terms of the incontinent woman "having a world," "losing a world" and "replacing a world." By having a world, I mean the woman's pre-diagnostic existence, that is her life before her ordeal began in terms of her everyday outlook and behaviors. By losing a world I mean to point to the assault that incontinence tends to have, namely, the person feels like their world of meaning that they once knew, lived and loved has been radically undermined and becomes something unpleasantly harsh and otherwise. Finally, by replacing a world, I mean the fact that every woman suffering from incontinence has to generate a new outlook and set of behaviors as a response to the assault on their everyday world.

Having a World

Like anyone, the typical woman who gets incontinence has what Erving Goffman called "a 'home world'—a way of life and a round of activities taken for granted until the point of" (Goffman, 1961, p. 12) realizing that she has the incontinence on a fairly regular basis. It is this world that gives the woman direction to her life and a feeling of safety and security.[1] Once the process of knowing herself as having frequent incontinence, that she for example "leaks," she begins to have to grapple with a strikingly different, if not harsher personal and social existence. In effect, it is her universe, her world of meanings, that begins to "leak." In her way of experiencing herself, especially her body, this may feel like she is going through a personal and social death, one that demands a reorganization of her way of being-in-the-world. Regardless of the type, incontinence which is not easily if at all medically correctable may feel like a form of imprisonment.

As sociologist Anthony Giddens noted, to fashion a world that one feels safe and secure in, where one is not threatened by say death anxiety (e.g., social death) requires more than simply consciously maintained propositional beliefs. Rather the most important, constituent element necessary for fashioning a world is engaged activity, what Giddens calls routines. By routinization Giddens means "the habitual, taken-for-granted character of the vast bulk of the activities of day-to-day life" (Giddens, 1984, p. 376). The importance of routines says Giddens is that it "is vital to the psychological mechanisms whereby a sense of trust or ontological security is sustained in the daily activities of social life," and "is integral…to the continuity of the personality of the agent, as he or she moves along the path of daily activities" (ibid., p. 60). Routines promote a sense of autonomy and integration in that it is through them that the person tends to experience the world as a place that can be controlled and understood and most importantly, effective decisions and interventions can be made. Moreover, there is generally a profound, generalized emotional involvement in the routines of daily life that connects a person to routines. That is, a routine allows the person to move relatively easily and securely in the world without being overwhelmed by death anxiety and the like. Routinization also diminishes the unconscious bases of anxiety. It is the channeling, organization and evasion of such primal tensions and diffuse anxiety that Giddens claims is one of the main motivations of human behavior.

Ontological security originates from one's home world in that it developed early in life by caregivers who create predictable and caring routines which promote adequate anxiety-controlling mechanisms in the child. Ontological security refers to the individuals "confidence or trust that the natural and social world are as they appear to be, including the basic existential parameters of self and social identity" (ibid., p. 376). This confidence and trust is lodged in a person's capacity to predict events and to control both himself and immediate situation. Following R.D. Laing, by ontological security I mean a person's sense of his presence in the world as real, alive, whole, and in a temporal sense, continuous. Says Laing, such a basically ontologically secure person will engage all challenges of life, social, ethical, spiritual, biological from a fundamentally firm and robust sense of his own and other people's inner reality and identity (Laing, 1962, p. 41). Such a person has trust in his own self-efficacy and his ability to influence the world he lives in. This is in marked contrast to an ontologically insecure person, such as the woman who loses her world. Such a person in her everyday life feels more unreal than real, more dead than alive. She may feel precariously separated from the rest of the world, so that her identity, integration and autonomy are always uncertain. She lacks the experience of her own temporal continuity and she may not possess an overriding sense of personal consistency and cohesiveness. She may feel more insubstantial than substantial, and unable to assume that the stuff she is made of is genuine, good, valuable (ibid., pp. 44–45). It is this kind of radical ontological insecurity, with its attendant reduction of autonomy and integration, that in part constitutes the woman's incontinent experience of losing her home world.

Thus, the continent woman has a rich involving personal and social existence, a meaningful world that sustains her. Put differently, such a woman has a world of, for example, love and work which is saturated with meaning. What happens when this continent world gives way to incontinence, when, the world she knew, lived and loved gives way to incontinence, a kind of assault on identity, autonomy and integration. It is to this subject that we turn to.

Losing a World

As Sinclair and Ramsay aptly summarize the matter,

> incontinent women are burdened with anxieties and feelings of embarrassment and shame and they live in constant fear that others will discover their condition. Women's sexual function and relationships with their partners are significantly affected by their incontinence thus augmenting their feelings of low self-confidence. Furthermore, major depression has been shown to be more common in incontinent women, adding to the cycle of low self-esteem, increased social withdrawal and, ultimately, a reduction in quality of life.
>
> (Sinclair & Ramsay, 2011, p. 147)[2]

Indeed, becoming incontinent presents a huge impediment for a woman to have a flourishing life.

In particular, says Sinclair and Ramsay, there are relationship difficulties, sexual function difficulties, exercise and sport difficulties, employment difficulties, travel and vacation difficulties and sleep difficulties.

Relationship Difficulties

From my clinical experience and research findings, many women who become incontinent view their intimate relationships as being diminished due to their condition. In particular, they feel anxious, if not hyper-vigilant about giving off an unpleasant smell and urine leakage and cannot easily relax, including in the bedroom (see below). In its extreme this can lead to a lack of stability and avoidance in their marriage or relationship with their significant other, even divorce or separation. Citing one study, Sinclair and Ramsay provide an illuminating quotation from an incontinent woman: "I become nervous and cannot actually relax. I am anxious about smelling bad and urine leakage when we are closely intimate" (ibid., p. 145). One woman who I saw in psychotherapy completely avoided intimate contact with her live-in boyfriend because she was so afraid of giving off a bad smell and/or urine leakage. She would spray the bathroom or bedroom respectively to conceal her "dirty truth" as she called it.

Sexual dysfunction, say Sinclair and Ramsay, is a fairly common complaint among women with urinary incontinence. This can include decreased desire, anorgasmia (difficulty getting an orgasm or sexual arousal) and dyspareunia (painful intercourse). Such symptoms as leaking during intercourse, embarrassment and depression are fairly common. One study cited by Sinclair and Ramsay indicated that women suffering from urge incontinence experienced greater difficulties with sexual incontinence than women with stress incontinence.

Exercise and Sport difficulties

As a result of their fear and anxiety, incontinent women may relinquish or seriously reduce the amount of exercise and sport they participate in for they are worried and troubled about others becoming aware of their condition. They thus relinquish the opportunity to stay more fit and involve themselves in social interaction. It is worth noting, according to Sinclair and Ramsay, that women with mixed incontinence often judge their urine leakage to be a greater inhibitor to exercise than those suffering from pure stress or urge incontinence. This was interpreted by these women as having to cope with both urinary leakage during exercise and having to locate a toilet immediately (ibid.). As a result of not exercising and overall engaging in a more inactive lifestyle, incontinent women can become overweight or obese. This can prevent them from having surgery for their condition until they lose weight, though they fear exercise and therefore have to delay such surgery, a kind of vicious cycle or endless thicket of problems.

Employment Difficulties

Women can have a very hard time in the work context, for example, symptoms of urinary incontinence can cause occupational inhibition as a consequence of worries regarding feeling wet and smelling of urine. Such anxiety, says Sinclair and Ramsay, can contribute to their reported loss of focus and concentration, loss of ability to adequately perform physical tasks, and disruption of work for toilet breaks. Such limitations influence their general work effectiveness as well as their self-confidence and self-efficacy. Studies have shown that urinary incontinence is indeed fairly common in the work context, and the more severe the condition the more often it happens. Sometimes this has led to such women not going to work due to their fear and anxiety of the obnoxious symptoms of their condition.

Travel and Vacation Difficulties

Traveling or going on vacation can be a particularly anxiety-ridden time for incontinent women. For example, says Sinclair and Ramsay, such women often feel reluctance to visit new places and worry that there will be no toilets nearby or that there will be no toilet accommodations at all. Lining up at public toilets may be particularly anxiety-producing, just as traveling on public facilities where there are no toilets can become highly agitating if not traumatic. These concerns, says Sinclair and Ramsay, are more frequent in women suffering from an overactive bladder, as the worry of urgency and urge incontinence without access to a toilet worsens the condition, leading to a vicious cycle and endless thicket of problems. As a result of all of the aforementioned, incontinent women may well choose to stay home and avoid traveling away from the relative comfort of their home world.

Sleep Difficulties

As a result of their condition, says Sinclair and Ramsay, incontinent women may have to get up a number of times during the night thus interfering in their getting enough high-quality sleep. With an overactive bladder they may not make it to the bathroom and have an accident, such as wetting their bed, enuresis, or being incontinent on the way to the bathroom. In addition to sleep deprivation there is the real possibility of the incontinent woman, especially when older, to falling and breaking the neck of femur (the area right below the ball of the hip joint), creating a range of medical problems and sometimes even death. Women may feel unease if they are suffering from stress incontinence, if they leak in bed such as when changing position or coughing or sneezing. Moreover, says Sinclair and Ramsay, wearing night pads can be quite uncomfortable and a source of irritation to the skin which can negatively impact the quality of sleep.

Quality of Life Difficulties

It is no surprise that the quality of life of women suffering from urinary incontinence can be profound, that is, says Sinclair and Ramsay, as a result of their condition they are prone to feel lower self-confidence and reduced self-efficacy, feeling mortified and embarrassed and unappealing to others. It is therefore to be expected that women suffering from urinary incontinence are vulnerable to the development of depression. Indeed, one study cited by Sinclair and Ramsay, reported that urinary incontinent women were about three times more likely to suffer from depression than continent women, a finding that fits well with the aforementioned interference in the urinary incontinent woman's quality of life. Such downward spiraling of aspects of their quality of life becomes a fertile breeding ground for the development of a range of neurotic conflicts, problems in living and sometimes psychiatric morbidity, including vulnerability to major depression, depending how the aforementioned limitations on their everyday life are managed. To make matters worse, the depressed incontinent woman, or the incontinent woman in general, may be less likely to convey her symptoms to her doctor feeling too uncomfortable, embarrassed or overwhelmed.

Thus, incontinent women have to endure a radical rupture to the life they lived prior to their condition becoming a longstanding problematic one. It is this losing of a world that I want to focus on. That is, the incontinent woman's near entire social existence has to be modified for they are usually totally unprepared for the situation that they find themselves. In the language of Giddens, such an extreme situation or "critical situation" as he calls it, fundamentally involves "circumstances of radical disjuncture of an unpredictable kind which affect substantial numbers of individuals, situations that threaten or destroy the certitudes of institutionalized routines" (Giddens, 1984, p. 16). With such a sustained assault on the incontinent woman's agency and pre-diagnosis routines that underpinned her ontological security, the woman is inundated with disorganizing affects and intense social death anxiety. This condition makes it nearly impossible to maintain her autonomy and integration or any kind of coherent narrative of self-identity. Trapped in a maze of grotesque happenings, the woman's options are greatly limited and she is often without hope of ever feeling "whole" or "normal" again.

Replacing a World

To some extent the way that the incontinent woman adjusts to her condition, as described above, is an attempt to replace her pre-incontinent existence with a liveable life as an incontinent woman. Thus, the deployment of tactics like avoidance of intimate relationships, including sexual contact, avoidance of exercise and sport, work restriction, social withdrawal when it comes to travel and vacations and avoiding wetting herself by disruption when it comes to sleep. Indeed, for a long time, women have coped with their condition with absorbent pads, by carrying an extra set of clothes, catheters, drainage bags, odor-control products, toilet aids etc. (Smith & Smith, 1987, p. 13) or as I said, by avoiding social settings and remaining at home. My claim is that a woman can better manage her condition and learn the art of "living well with incontinence," what I am calling replacing a world (Pettit & Chen, 2021, p. 113).[3]

Perhaps the main thrust of living well with incontinence is to resist feeling humiliated. Following philosopher Richard Rorty, by humiliation I mean, what people say to themselves:

Now that I have believed and desired this, I can never be what I hoped to be, what I thought I was. The story I have been telling myself about myself—my picture of myself as honest, or loyal, or devout—no longer makes sense. I no longer have a self to make sense of. There is no world in which I can picture myself living, because there is no vocabulary in which I can tell a coherent story about myself.

(Rorty, 1989, p. 179)

In other words, women who feel humiliated in this way (or approximately this way), are not willing and able to integrate events which occurred in their every lives and sort them into the ongoing story about the self (a narrative of self-identity). Such humiliation "shatters all molds designed to contain a unified and irreproachable image of the self" (Langer, 1991, p. 77), and for the incontinent woman to revamp her self-concept, increase her self-esteem and better navigate her everyday life, she must have the will and ability to create a different world of meanings for herself, one that takes into consideration her incontinence not as a badge of shame. Put differently, such subversion of one's identity and damaged self-esteem undermines the woman's ontological security, that all important sense of continuity and order in events. As Giddens has pointed out, when one's ontological security is severely assaulted, chaos breaks in, but "this chaos is not just disorganization, but the loss of a sense of the very reality of things and of other persons" (Giddens, 1991, p. 36). Psychologically speaking, says Giddens, this chaos can be viewed as "dread" in Kierkegaard's sense, being overwhelmed by anxieties that reach to the very roots of one's coherent self-identity (ibid., p. 37). Thus, the loss of everyday contexts for action and meaning, the loss of a sense of membership, the inability of individuals to assert and affirm identity, is a situation of intense psychic and social instability (Weinstein & Platt, 1973). Maintaining the continuity and coherence of one's narrative of self-identity in such a context is thus extremely difficult, if not impossible. However, in my view, those women with the emotional and intellectual resources tend to be more successful at salvaging whatever they can of their pre-incontinent self, and thus to some extent can avoid the feeling of extreme humiliation and degradation.

By replacement world I mean a new set of routines—both attitudinal (i.e., a revised narrative of self-identity) and behavioral that help to give a degree of order and direction to the incontinent woman's life in what she regards as an extreme situation. A replacement world includes a new reference group—a group whose beliefs, attitudes and behaviors provide a standard against which they compare and orient themselves. A replacement world also involves a new set of roles— different behaviors displayed in connection with the incontinent woman's new inferior social position as she construes it. Thus, a replacement world gives the incontinent woman a minimal sense of control, self-esteem and ontological security, and helps them to continue to press on in her struggle to live a flourishing life despite her disability. What does this affect-integrating, meaning-giving, action-guiding replacement world look like?

It should be clear that today there are some relatively effective ways to manage urinary incontinence. Behavior therapies, medications, and surgical procedures can significantly reduce, maybe even eliminate urinary leakage and help a woman regain bladder control (Pettit & Chen, 2021, p.113). However, there are additional practical everyday strategies, emotional, intellectual and pragmatic resources that can reduce the anxiety-ridden risk, and change and adapt one's everyday environment (ibid.). An incontinent woman has some control over her condition but there are other lifestyle and other factors that she does not have control over, and there lies the rub.

Reducing Risk of an Anxiety-Ridden Accident

The practical strategies I will be mentioning drawn from Pettit & Chen (2021) are illustrative and not a complete list of resources that relate to changing one's lifestyle to a healthier one, for the incontinent woman.

1   Add additional fiber to your diet since constipation is a pertinent contributor to incontinence. "Keeping your bowel movements soft and regular permits urine to freely flow, and it reduces the strain that is placed on a woman's pelvic floor muscles" (ibid., p. 114).
2   Shun bladder irritants. This involves reducing food and beverages that irritate the bladder, and therefore one is less likely to be incontinent. For instance, drinking a lot of coffee will often make a woman go to the bathroom more often.
3   Maintain adequate liquid intake (e.g., about eight 8 ounce glasses of water!). As Pettit and Chen note, drinking too much fluid can make a woman urinate more often. But not drinking enough can lead to an unhealthy concentration of waste in your urine, which can irritate a woman's bladder and cause an upsurge of urgency and frequency.
4   Lose excess weight. If you are overweight, losing excessive pounds can help diminish overall pressure on your bladder, pelvic floor muscles and related nerves. Even losing about 71/2 pounds of body weight can reduce symptoms associated with incontinence.
5   Physical exercise. Doing 30 minutes of physical activity a few days a week cannot only improve fitness, but it strengthens muscles, helps reduce weight and preserves independence and autonomy in older women. The important point is that "exercise can reduce the risk of incontinence caused by restricted mobility or difficulty in managing zippers and buttons" (ibid., p. 115). Regular exercise also fends off depression as is well-known, and for middle-aged women depression is often associated with incontinence. Pettit and Chen point out that for women who have urine leakage during

exercise they may want to use a urethral or vaginal insert, which aids in preventing leakage. Some women, they say, have effectively used super tampons or a diaphragm for support.

6   Avoid smoking. Smoking can lead to a serious chronic cough, which can worsen symptoms of stress incontinence. By cease smoking, coughing is reduced and this further reduces the pressure the coughing places on a woman's bladder and pelvic floor muscles.[4]

Changing and Adapting to Your Environment

As Pettit and Chen note, if you have difficulty getting to the bathroom on time due to restricted mobility, such as arthritis or recent hip surgery, engaging in making a few changes within your dwelling may help ward off incontinent episodes such as:

1   Situate your bedroom close to the bathroom.
2   Maintain a well-lit path to the bathroom free of impediments that may slow you down or cause an accident like falling on the way to the toilet.
3   Putting in an elevated toilet so that it's simpler to sit down and get up.
4   Putting in grab bars to assist you getting on and off the toilet.
5   Keeping a bedpan or urinal close bye in your bedroom.
6   Having a portable toilet nearby if your only bathroom is up or down an unwieldy flight of stairs.
7   Consulting with an Occupational Therapist can help the incontinent woman, old or young, with the consequences of aging, sickness or injury in the effective management and navigation of their everyday lives.
8   Proper clothing. If you have an overactive bladder and you go to the bathroom often, it is useful to decrease the number of articles of clothing you wear. Obviously, dressing in a number of layers can make it more hard going to get to the toilet on time.
9   Engaging the outside world. It is imperative that one not give in to anxiety and engage the social world for this reduces feelings of isolation and depression that often accompany incontinence. Staying connected to people is important for obvious reasons.
10 Behavior therapists such as pelvic floor muscle training and bladder training can assist a woman to gain better control over her bladder so she can endure a work meeting or a movie or a play without having to go to the bathroom.

Pettit & Chen suggest that there are other fairly obvious suggestions a woman can deploy when she goes out of the house into the everyday social world. They are worth mentioning.

1   Carry needed supplies with you. When leaving home, take a sufficient number of incontinence pads or protective undergarments with you. Thus, if an accident occurs the woman can feel confident that she can discretely cope with the situation without having to go home immediately.
2   Some sensible women carry a change of clothing with them. A bulky sweater wrapped around your waist can be helpful in case of an emergency. Carrying a zippered plastic bag, says Pettit and Chen, to place soiled clothing until you arrive home can also be useful.
3   Search out your destination. What this boils down to is familiarizing yourself with the locations of the toilets at the place you are going to. Something as simple as sitting on the isle at a movie or a house of worship makes getting to the toilet much easier.

Sexuality and Incontinence

As Pettit and Chen note, leaking during intercourse can be a very distressing moment for a woman, this is especially the case with women with stress incontinence. In that instance,

> they leak when the man's penis presses against the urethra and bladder upon initial penetration. With women with urge incontinence, urine leakage may be more unpredictable, though it often happens during orgasm and in greater volume than women with stress incontinence.
>
> (ibid., p. 120)

Needless to say, with this on one's mind, it is hard to relax during sex. Below is a list of practical suggestions that Pettit and Chen say a woman can deploy to increase her confidence in herself and her ability for free, flowing and unrestrained sexual expression.

1   Increase and deepen the conversation between you and your partner in order to maximize the partner's empathy for your condition and surrounding anxiety. Open communication is the watchword for sex on the rigorously sexual level.
2   Expand your definition of sex to centrally include various kinds of touching if sexual intercourse is too unwieldy.

3   A woman is less likely to leak if the position during sex is more comfortable for her, allowing her to concentrate on the pleasuring rather than her anxiety about urinary incontinence. In general, says Pettit and Chen, women on top often provides better pelvic muscle control, just as rear entry may reduce pressure on her bladder.

4   Empty your bladder prior to sex and avoid drinking any liquids about an hour before sex.

5   Use a diaphragm. "Because of where a diaphragm sits in the female pelvis, it can provide support to the bladder and urethra and help prevent leakage during sexual intercourse" (ibid, p. 121).

6   Do pelvic floor muscle exercises (Kegels), which can strengthen a woman's pelvic floor muscles and limit leakage.

7   If you are anxious about wetness, be prepared by having towels near-bye or using disposable pads on your bed.

8   Having a sense of humor and practicing positive thinking are particularly helpful in reducing a woman's anxiety (this is easier said than done)

9   Finding the right doctor who you can work with is essential.

Final Comments: the Challenges of Female Incontinence

I have deliberately structured the aforementioned material on losing and replacing a world in a very practical form (hence, mainly drawing from four gynecological clinical practitioners), so that the reader can get a nitty-gritty, nuts and bolts understanding of what adult urine incontinent women may distressingly go through each day. In this concluding section, I want to briefly deepen the analysis of the problems in living that these women face.

Perhaps the main problem for the incontinent woman is protecting her "inner self", such that she recognizes herself as the same woman she was prior to the onset of her incontinence (i.e., there is a sense of biographical continuity). This is no easy task for her symptoms, and the everyday lifestyle changes she has to engage in to best manage the symptoms, feel all-encompassing. Thus, the incontinent woman's struggle is a moral struggle aimed at maintaining her integration, autonomy and humanity in a manner that at least calls to mind her pre-incontinent existence. By integration I mean that her sense of self, the parts of herself are felt to be an interdependent, interconnected and interrelated whole. By autonomy I mean mainly decision-making. And by humanity, I mean having agency to be the kind of person one wants to be without interfering in other's well-being. All of this requires that the incontinent woman remembers that she has a degree of attitudinal freedom as she confronts her new circumstances. In other words, she has to be mindful of the fact that to protect herself from self-alienation from her body requires reorganizing her self-concept and self-esteem in a manner that reflects her agency.

This entails coming to terms with the fact that to some extent, her incontinent symptoms reflect the organism's breakdown, such that the body can be experienced as a stranger to oneself. Where one remembers having an intact body, now the incontinent woman has one that literally and metaphorically leaks. This is a process that reflects the fact that the typical incontinent woman enters into a very complex and deeply troubling relationship with her body, especially when the aging process has a strong interpretive grip on her consciousness. It is a situation where she feels the horror of being an ego/self and non-ego/not self, familiar and estranged, existing and not existing, at the same time. This means that her prior to incontinence existence when she regarded herself as an acceptable, if not lovable and integrated person is called into question, at least to some extent. The gist of the aforementioned is the fact that the incontinent woman may feel herself to be young and vibrant but her body tells her otherwise, that is, there can be an alienating sense of exhaustion or worse, at the notion of having to carry on living and being herself.

The aforementioned suggests why the typical incontinent woman sometimes has a kind of narcissistic sadness, which can turn into a depressive reaction or worse. This is because unlike say arthritis, the symptoms of incontinence cut deeply into the self (i.e., into a woman's "womanliness") in a way that other medical conditions usually don't. Without being able to maintain much, or any narcissistic satisfaction associated with one's pre-incontinent life, the incontinent woman is left trying to revive her intact and enlivened sense of self when she felt better about herself as an integrated being. Indeed, as French phenomenological philosopher Maurice Merleau-Ponty noted, we are first and foremost "body subjects," that is, all of human consciousness must be comprehended via our bodies, their way of relating to her bodies, and the world they create and inhabit. Emotions are crucial to this sense of "embodiment," that is, emotions like self-loathing are primary elements of our existence that always work through our bodies, that much more so for the incontinent woman (Langdridge, 2015). For example, our relation to our body is in part, a reflection of the unconscious internalization of socio-cultural norms and prohibitions about what constitutes the ideal body image, beauty and intactness, and this can have dire consequences for the deteriorating incontinent woman when she reflects on her situation. Put differently, the way we experience our body and the world, in this case, our relationship to other bodies, are inevitably connected. To some extent, we view our body the way we fantasize others see us, which can be a psychologically rough moment for the incontinent woman when her fantasy is accusative ("I am broken", "my plumbing is defective").

Another way of stating the aforementioned is that the woman's ontological security is undermined. It is this jarring alienation from herself as an intact continent woman, that can make the incontinent woman feel unwilling and unable to "lean in" to the future. This can be a fertile breeding ground for the development of a wide range of neurotic and other conflicts, for there is some painful reality to her anguish. After all, the incontinent woman cannot run away from her broken body, she cannot jettison herself out of her skin, no matter how much she aspires to doing so.

Thus, the body that once effectively mediated her relationship between her and the world now becomes the body that estranges her from the world and space. Through the body's undeniably downwardly modified functionality, it can lead to a real and metaphorical sense of imprisonment. The incontinent woman's relationship to her significantly diminished bodily subjectivity promotes the sense that the world has become a mean-spirited adversary. In its extreme, such a response to the perceived hostile world calls to mind R.D. Laing's description of "petrification," a protective response to the upsurge of ontological insecurity (a lack of trust in one's physical existence and continuity of the world) associated with schizophrenia, such that the incontinent woman switches off and disconnects herself from the everyday world, as if a stone, and thus feels safely depersonalized (Langdridge, 2015).

The "dissociation of the ego" is especially manifest when a typical incontinent woman has to contend with her chronic condition: "If only this god damned body would leave me in peace." When one has to surmount chronic incontinence one distressingly relates to one's body as an unavoidable and extreme "materialization and substantiation," that is, she is "thrown" into a mode of self-relating that experiences the body as "*more* mass and *less* energy" (Améry, 1994, p. 39). This "heaviness of being" can feel as if one were strapped to a dying beast. This is in contrast to one's former mode of self-relating, the "lightness of being" associated with youth and health, that is, one's pre-incontinent existence. The incontinent woman is again caught in the paradox of becoming a stranger to herself through her chronic condition while also becoming more herself as an embodied being. As

Améry aptly puts it, "I [the incontinent woman] am myself *through* my body and *against* it" (as it is an adversary) while in earlier life, "I was myself when I was young *without* my body and *with* it" (ibid., p. 40). In other words, the incontinent woman's body is simultaneously experienced in terms of its gradual reduction of energy and self-efficacy and its gradual enlargement as a mere material entity and site of inadequacy, horridly signifying that she is an organism getting ready to eternally rest.

Without a cultivated imagination, the incontinent woman is unable to have the sensibility to adequately appreciate what is beautiful and pleasing in the world, and in herself, which includes one's sexual partner. Such a "disordered imagination" of being unable to properly visualize and generate imagery, including mentally stimulating purposeful action in a context-sensitive manner, such as occurs in autism and schizophrenia, is disastrous, especially in the bedroom. What is needed is an "aesthetic attitude," a specific way of experiencing or focusing on people and objects, one that is characterized by a heightened receptiveness, a sharpened reactivity to what is going on inside and outside oneself, similar to how a great actress engages her work (Marcus & Marcus, 2011, p. 213).[5]

As psychoanalyst Donald Winnicott argued, the goal of psychoanalysis is to transform

> the patient from a state of not being able to play into a state of being able to play....It is in playing and only in playing that the individual child or adult is able to be creative and to use the whole personality, and it is only in being creative that the individual discovers the self.
>
> (Winnicott, 1971, p. 10)

Moreover, "it is the creative apperception more than anything else that makes the individual feel that life is worth living" (ibid., p. 65). Indeed, there is an important moral truth embedded in Winnicott's psychological observations, that "man defines himself by his make-believe as well as by his sincere impulses" (Camus, 1955, p. 11). It is precisely by tapping the incontinent woman's capacity to creatively/imaginatively "play," similar to how a great stage actor "plays" to her fellow thespians and audience, that the conditions of possibility for an erotically-charged, emotionally satisfying experience between an incontinent and continent partner in the bedroom are created.

In conclusion, what seems to distinguish the incontinent woman who better manages her condition is her overall attitude towards her incontinence. To the extent that she believes that her condition is surmountable, that she is similar to how she was before her diagnosis, she can learn to anticipate problems in living and adapt accordingly to her circumstances in say love and work. This is no easy matter, for it requires the woman to constantly balance her needs of her inner self and the demands of her condition. Put differently, she must decide how far she will go to cater to her condition before she relinquishes her autonomy and dignity, before she gives the incontinence too much of herself. This often requires testing the vast number of choices which she has to make against her values and interests and thereby cut the wide range of problems down to manageable size. Compared to the poorly adapted incontinent woman, she feels more able to balance how much of herself she could surrender to her condition and still maintain the rudiments of her autonomy, integration and humanity. Perhaps most significantly, the well-adapted incontinent woman has a narrative of self-identity that gives her an ability to make some sense out of her condition, gives direction to her life vis a vis her condition and strengthens her sense of personhood (Giddens, 1991, pp. 52–54). As Giddens point out, such a woman has a more-or-less coherent narrative of self-identity that allows her to create a "protective cocoon" that "filters out" in the conduct of day to day life, many of the dangers and primal anxieties which often threaten the integrity of inner self. Such a person's ontological security is more securely anchored. The incontinent woman is thus willing and able to accept her integrity as worthwhile and there is adequate self-esteem to sustain a sense of self as "alive," within the scope of reflexive control, rather than having an inert quality of things in the object world (e.g., petrification). In contrast, the incontinent woman who is not able to adapt to her condition, not able to generate a replacement world, she is fated to live in a nightmarish state of brokenness, embarrassment and anxiety.

Notes

1 An earlier version in a different context of some of this material in this chapter can be found in Marcus (2019).
2 I have drawn liberally from gynecological clinicians Sinclair and Ramsay's (2011) excellent review article in this section, losing a world.
3 I have liberally drawn from gynecological clinicians Pettit & Chen's (2021) excellent practical guide to managing incontinence, in this section, replacing a world.
4 There are numerous self-care products for incontinence such as bladder control pads, pull-ons, adult briefs and skin care and odor products, See Pettit and Chen (2021, p. 116) for details.

5 The so-called "sapiosexuals" have rediscovered the long-known truth, as the *New York Times* titled its article, "the hottest body part is the brain" (North, 2017, p. A18).

References

Améry, J. (1994). *On Aging: Revolt and Resignation.* JD. Barlow (Trans.). Bloomington: Indiana University Press (Original work published in 1968).

Camus, A. (1955). *The Myth of Sisyphus and Other essays.* New York: Knopf.

Debus, G., and R. Kastner (2015). Psychosomatic aspects of urinary incontinence. *Geburtsh Frauenheilk*, 75, 165–169.

Giddens, A. (1984). *The Constitution of Society.* Berkeley: University of California Press.

Giddens, A. (1991). *Modernity and Self-Identity.* Stanford: Stanford University Press.

Goffman, E. (1961). *Asylums.* Garden City: Anchor Books.

Kuoch, K.L.J., G.S. Hebbard, H.E. O'Connell, D.W. Austin, and S.R. Knowles (2019). Urinary and faecal incontinence: psychological factors and management recommendations. *New Zealand Medical Association*, 132 (1503), 25–33.

Laing, R.D. (1962). Ontological Insecurity. In H.M. Ruitenbeck (ed.) *Psychoanalysis and Existential Philosophy*, New York: E.P. Dutton and Company, 38–52.

Langdridge, D. (2015). *Existential Counseling and Psychotherapy.* London: Sage.

Langer, L.L. (1991). *Holocaust Testimonies.* New Haven: Yale University Press.

Marcus, P. (2019). *The Psychoanalysis of Overcoming Suffering. Flourishing Despite Pain.* London: Routledge.

Marcus, P. with G. Marcus (2011). *Theatre as Life: Practical Wisdom Drawn from Great Acting Teachers, Actors and Actresses.* Milwaukee: Marquette University Press.

North, A. (2017). The Hottest Body Part? For a Sapiosexual, It's the Brain. *New York Times*, June 13, p. A18.

Pettit, P.D., & Chen, A.H. (2021). *Mayo Clinic on Incontinence. Strategies and treatments for improving bladder and bowel control.* Rochester: Mayo Clinic Press.

Rorty, R. (1989). *Contingency, Irony and Solidarity.* Cambridge: Cambridge University Press.

Sinclair, A.J., and Ramsay, I.N. (2011). The psychosocial impact of urinary incontinence in women. *Royal College of Obstetricians and Gynecologists*, 13, 143–148.

Smith, P.S. & Smith, L.J. (1987). *Continence and Incontinence. Psychological Approaches to Development and Treatment.* London: Croom Helm.

Tranquility (2016). https://tranquilityproducts.com.

Weinstein, F. & Platt, G. (1973). *Psychoanalytic Sociology.* Baltimore: John Hopkins University Press.

Winnicott, D.W. (1971). *Playing and Reality.* London: Tavistock.

Chapter 4

Toilet Cursing

Cursing, swearing or trash-talking, often euphemistically called "potty mouth" (Haslam, 2012, p. 93) has a number of important psychological and social functions in individual and collective life respectively. In this chapter, I will mainly focus on the so-called "anal-phase" related cursing for that is the form that cursing tends to take. Scatological means relating to or characterized by an attentiveness in excrement and excretion as in scatological humor. Scatological language is regarded as a universal phenomenon, though what constitutes scatological in a particular culture is context-dependent and setting-specific (Mohr, 2013; Haslam, 2012; Gregory and James, 2009).[1] For example, people call each other (or sometimes themselves) *asshole, shit or shit-ass*, or say to someone *piss-off, you are pissing me off, don't take the piss out of me*, or they reference the penis, such as *dick, cock, willy* or *prick* and urination usually in a derogatory manner (Haslam, 2012). There are many other ways these words and phrases are used depending on the era, society and sub-group one is in, though for the most part, most toilet cursing in our society/era has an anal theme to it, with faecal references being most often used, followed by flatulence and urinary terms (ibid.). The word shit for instance can be used in a wide variety of taboo and sanitized, literal and non-literal anally animated ways as is common knowledge (ibid). Thus, this chapter will discuss the role of scatological in the extreme, as in telephone scatalogia, *coprolalia* ("shit speech" as in Tourette's and other medical conditions), and *caprophagia* (literally "shit eating").[2] However, the focus will be on what the experience of such toilet cursing is for the ordinary person who says it (less the "mentally ill" such as the psychotic who engages in caprophagia), whether it is articulated to others or privately to oneself.

Psychoanalytic Musings on Toilet Cursing

Not surprisingly, the psychoanalytic story about toilet cursing begins in the anal stage. In instinct theory, the anal stage denotes the period of

DOI: 10.4324/9781003219705-4

psychosexual development roughly between a year and a half and three years. As Freud noted, this is the moment the child's pleasurable preoccupation is transferred from the mouth and orality, to the anus and anality (Akhtar, 2009). That is, the child's main pleasure is derived by the movement of feces through the anal mucous membrane, such that the anus, anal sphincter, defecation and feces are what matter most to the child. The idea here, continues Akhtar, is that the child derives great pleasure from withholding feces with the fantasized aspiration that greater pleasure can be attained from the mucous membrane. This focus on feces is the basis for anal eroticism. The child also fantasizes about his aggressively jettisoning or expelling his feces. This is the basis for anal sadism. Another psychological shift happens when the child is toilet trained, in an effort to socialize him. The child morphs his preoccupation with feces and his body ego (the aspect of the ego that evolves out of self-perceptions of the body), to the parental caregivers, especially the main parental caregiver, usually the mother in our society. This shift has been described as the move from anal auto-eroticism to anal object relations (ibid). As Freud (1917) noted feces becomes equated with affectionate gift-giving, "look mommy what a big poop I did."[3] As is well known, a typical toddler vacillates between these two extremes, an expression of anal ambivalence, as it is typically called (Akhtar, 2009). Thus anal-eroticism, anal-sadism and anal ambivalence are the key conceptual ports of entry into understanding toilet cursing, at least from the point of view of instinct theory, and for that matter most other psychoanalytic theories though these concepts are recast in less instinctual terms (i.e., object relations).

Of historical interest, at least in our society, is the "faecal stick" insinuated by Freud in his discussion of the anal phase (1918), and discussed by Karl Abraham (Akhtar, 2009). A "shit stick or stake" (sometimes with a small sponge attached to it) was used instead of toilet paper for anal hygiene and was a historical tool of material culture first initiated through Chinese and Japanese Buddhism. As Akhtar notes, Abraham's idea was that the faecal stick can be a psychological antecedent of the penis and this can conflate in the child's phantasy such that relinquishing feces is comparable to castration. Also, worth mentioning is that the child can phantasize a presumed unconscious equivalence among feces-penis-baby, which can be the conditions of possibility for the fantasy of anal birth and the sexual wishes for anal penetration by the father (an alleged common phantasy in children). Finally, says Akhtar, children don't easily give up their feces, a body product that they regard as intrinsic to whom they are, and thus, there is an inclination to retrieve the feces as a way of affirming their budding identity. Shit eating (caprophagia) and fecal smearing among little children in reality or phantasy are extreme manifestations. The aforementioned points inevitably have a major impact on the child's personality or character development, hence the famous anal character or personality which has been memorialized, or at least "recycled" in our era as the obsessive-compulsive personality.[4] Themes of "control" versus "compliance," and "retentiveness" versus "giving," are particularly noteworthy with regards to anal character development, as is emphasized in object relations theory (ibid, p. 14). For Freud, the anal character is characterized by orderliness, parsimony and obstinance: "Orderly covers the notion of bodily cleanliness, as well as conscientiousness in carrying out small duties and trustworthiness. Parsimony may appear in the exaggerated form of avarice; and obstinacy can go over into defiance" (Freud, 1908, p. 169). Overall, says Akhtar, there has been a "Cultural abhorrence of anal matters," leading to a "'heuristic repression' of the anal phase" in psychoanalytic literature (though there have been a few exceptions) especially in terms of learning about ourselves from toilet practices, our main concern in this book, and in this chapter, from anal-animated cursing (Akhtar, 2009, p. 14).

Toilet cursing can be a manifestation of anal eroticism, what Shengold (1988) calls "anal narcissism," what boils down to a regressive way of being-in-the-world such that the person is governed by the anal-sadistic organization and the correlated diminution of mature-like ego to body ego (a much more primitive state of bodily sensations). As Shengold notes,

> the anal narcissistic defense... acts as a kind of emotional and sensory closeable door that serves to control the largely murderous and cannibalistic primal affects derived from the destructive and from the perverse sexual drives of early life. This "door" operates along the body ego mode... of the control of the anal sphincter.
>
> (Shengold, 1988, p. 24)

What this means is that the person's way of relating to value and meaning, especially to others, is to make them into "undifferentiated *stuff*," in other words, "excretable shit" (ibid.). Drawing from Karl Abraham, Shengold noted, "relationships become self-centered and hollow; people are reduced to things; values to stuff" (ibid., p. 76). Put simply then, from a psychoanalytic point of view, toilet cursing is a person's way of expressing aggressive and sexual wishes meant to do some kind of harm to the target of the outburst. This harm can be real or imagined, that is in the realm of phantasy. The harm that is wished for is to make the other person feel like shit, "the grey, the undifferentiated, the meaningless" (ibid., p. 39). This is largely based on the fact that shit has negative symbolic meanings in our society that most people grasp.

Symbolism of Excrement

In order to grasp the psychoanalytic functions of toilet cursing it is necessary to have a sense of the symbolism of excrement, for in our society toilet cursing almost always references one of the many symbolic meanings of excrement. Praeger (2007) aptly describes some of these symbolic meanings, meanings that resonate with psychoanalytic theory. A few examples are instructive.

First, excrement symbolizes the "lowness of the high" (ibid., p. 121). As Freud wrote, "it is far from being a simple matter to survey or describe the consequences involved in this way of treating the 'embarrassing trace on Earth,' of which the sexual and excretory functions may be considered its nucleus" (Freud, 1913, p. 6). What Freud is getting at has been known by scatological humorists for a long time, namely, as William Plank notes, shit "removes the props by which the self attempts to create and control its image [presentation of the self as Goffman calls it]: clothing, privacy, secrecy, composition of the face, and self-control" (Praeger, 2007, p. 122). In other words, when someone high in status is publicly revealed to be all too human in terms of his being an excreting animal, a complete person that he has attempted to conceal, the unmasking is not only humorous, but it is humbling, particularly when the person responds with embarrassment. A good example of a famous man who was tragically taken down in this manner was described by Milan Kundera in the *Unbearable Lightness of Being*. After the Second World War, says Praeger, Stalin's son Yakov was imprisoned by the Germans and held in a prison camp along with a bunch of British soldiers. Yakov had a habit of leaving a mess in the prisoners' collective latrine. The British officers were very angry, even if this was the excrement of the son of the one of the most powerful men in the world. The British soldiers attempted to discuss it with Yakov but he refused. They attempted to force him to clean the latrine but he refused. Finally, the dispute grew so unpleasant that Yakov insisted on a hearing with the camp arbiter. However, the arbiter would not devalue himself by discussing a topic so lowly. Yakov was humiliated, his pre-incarceration self-concept and self-esteem were seriously subverted. Cursing profusely to conceal his shame, he ran into the electrified fence, and died. In other words when Yakov's belief that his social position made his excrement exceptional was invalidated, he could not sustain his narrative of self-coherence. When the German arbiter refused to discuss the issue, Yakov had to face the contrary realization, that he was like everyone else. Yakov, says Praeger,

> was being judged, not for his role in the dramas of war, politics, power, or family, but for his pooh. The high of being the son of Stalin was destroyed by the lowness of pooh. Yakov could not live without the façade.
>
> (ibid., p. 123)

Toilet cursing, whether in a serious or humorous context, is geared to unmask a person's high and mighty presentation—his perceived hubris—so that he is situated on a level playing field of a complete human who is as much an animal as he is anything else. For many people, putting on a façade is fundamental to their presentation of self and when they are cut down to size by toilet cursing in reality or fantasy, the diminution is very satisfying to the unmasker and other observers. I am reminded of my patient who was going for an interview at a prestigious university for a teaching job and was very anxious about the interview. However, when he visualized the interviewer on the toilet, grunting away, he felt less intimidated by the authoritative "professorial big shot" as he called him who was judging his career fate.

Second, excrement symbolizes "the lowness of the low" (ibid., p. 123). Excrement is regarded by just about everyone as the lowest of the low in terms of substance and meaning. Therefore, anything that it gets connected to is correspondingly diminished in status. In the film *Chattahoochee*, says Praeger, a Korean War hero named Emmet Foley ends up in a psychiatric hospital where doctors seem more focused on humiliating their patients than in properly treating and caring for them. He revolts and is punished by being forced to sit on a hard object that should make his agony of boredom and pain worse, and then the inevitable finally happens: he first wets himself, and then he soils himself. In Foley's case the doctors were teaching him the harsh way that they had complete authoritative control over his physical and mental well-being (calling to mind Goffman's "total institution"). The fact that their "power extended to bodily functions make the low appear even lower" (ibid.). While I will be taking up this theme on excremental assault in the Nazi concentration camp in the last chapter, what is most important here is how someone who has been made powerless, or near powerless, can be made to feel even lower by the skillful use of excrement to demean and devalue. In the case of toilet cursing, to call someone who is already regarded as a failure in his own eyes, is to cut even more deeply into his sense of dignity. An abusive father who had mainly psychologically abused his under-functioning and truant son because he was a lousy student who also cut class from time to time, was called by his father "a little shit," and "the asshole" which the teenager told me in treatment made him feel even worse about himself and fueled his rage at his father. Cutting his nose off to spite his face (that is purposefully failing academically) was worth it to him he told me.

Third, excrement "makes a potent insult" (ibid., p. 124). The fact is that if you want to put a person down, insult them, excrement is the least ambiguous negative in our culture. This in part, because literally to most people it looks, smells and most people assume, tastes bad. Figuratively, it signifies the worst of anything, the worst appearance, smell or taste. It is thus not surprising that when one wants to insult another person, one draws on toilet cursing, on excremental language to convey one's negative sentiments. For example, one patient of mine told me that I was "a shit analyst." In other instances, like when a person says, "This tastes like shit," or "Today you played basketball like shit," the reference is either to an actual fecal manifestation or more likely, an abstract negative (ibid., p. 125). Perhaps the most poignant use of excrement as an insult was that to Jesus just before he was crucified and died on the cross. The public bathrooms of ancient Rome, says Praeger, supplied brine-soaked sponges on sticks for Romans to wipe their rear ends. In these "accounts of Jesus's cruci-fixion, Mark, Matthew, and John relate that the mocking crowd pushed a vinegar-soaked sponge into Jesus's face, smearing his face as a final indignity before his death" (in effect saying that what he preached was excrement) (ibid., p. 126). Toilet cursing can thus have various meanings including the target being linked to excrement lit-erally speaking, and/or, figuratively associated with the properties of excrement or defecating.[5]

Fourth, excrement symbolizes "contamination" (ibid., p. 127). It was Mary Douglas (1966) who famously engages with dirt as an extensive metaphor for anything that is symbolically polluting because it threatens established sociocultural categories, such as the division between males and females, human and animal, public and private. Dirt is an "offense against order," against categories that help promote social stability (it is "out of place," ibid., p. 44). It is, therefore, that which a society feels it needs to obliterate, conceal, or purify in order to preserve order. Sounds, smells, sights, objects or even people that cross boundaries threaten the purity of social categories and are causes of psychological and social unease. Thus, says Praeger, the concept of filth is profoundly enmeshed with ideas of class and hierarchy. The more you permit it out of its place, the less you are part of civilization. In our society that cherishes purity, "a filthy body implies a filthy soul. And no other filth is as filthy as poop. Out of place, it invites immediate and total condemnation" (Praeger, 2007, p. 127). Excrement, says Praeger, appears to have a supernatural-like ability to contaminate anything it touches, to such an extent that we will empty a hundred thousand gallons of water due to a few ounces of excrement lurking in a swimming pool (ibid., p. 128). Overreaction to excrement's contaminating presence, Praeger opines, appears to be more-or-less normative. For example, I remember an adult patient of mine telling me his worst memory of being jumped by three teens when he was about age 11, and in the fighting one of the teens found a piece of newspaper with dog excrement on it and smeared it into my patients face, freaking him out in disgust to this day.

Thus, toilet cursing can be so devastating to the victim because it is associated with the polluting that violates a core belief and value in the social system: social barrier crossing. "A polluting person is always in the wrong," he represents disorder because "dirt [shit] is essentially disorder" (Douglas, 1966, p. 2), and someone who is convincingly described that way sees himself that way too (ibid., p. 140). What makes toilet cursing with the contaminating theme so awful for the victim is that it is a variation on soul murder. It sucks the life out of them.

Fifth, embracing your own excrement can symbolize "contempt for others" (Praeger, 2007, p. 129). For example, take farting at someone, it tends to devalue the other, reduce his dignity and yet ironically, leaves the farter unharmed. Lyndon Johnson used to be quite matter of fact, defecate on the toilet and conduct his presidential duties in plain sight of visitors often embarrassing them in the extreme. In these instances, the record shows that Johnson felt that those who turned away in embarrassment or disgust were judged by him as faulty and flawed, as he felt utterly justified in his unusual way of conducting presidential business. The point is that toilet cursing can emphasize contempt for the other plain and simple, even though it is the curser who is behaving in a manner that you would expect most people to judge as unfairly discrediting, but the casual onlooker tends not to make such an attribution.

Sixth, excrement can symbolically "communicate protest" (ibid., p. 131). This is an all too familiar use of excrement. Toilet cursing can be a way of registering one's protest at injustice and the like. Data from hospitals, prisons and regional secure units have reported instances where fecal smearing occurred as a form of protest (ibid.,

132). Likewise, certain types of artistic creations that use excrement literally or figuratively, do so as a form of protest to what the artist perceives as societal oppressiveness. The great social critic and satirist comedian Lenny Bruce famously used toilet and other cursing in his acts. (By the way, Lenny Bruce died of a heroin overdose in 1966 while sitting on the toilet.) Toilet humor, and for that matter, toilet cursing than, can be an expression of inordinate frustration, powerlessness, negativity and vulnerability that is turned into its opposite through cursing.

Seventh, excrement, including toilet cursing, can represent "intimacy" (ibid., p. 140), as when a couple eliminate in front of each other or one of the partners uses foul anal animated language in a lighthearted (or not so lighthearted) manner. In other words, there is a close connection between intimacy and excretory honesty and integrity, and likewise, feeling uninhibited to use toilet cursing at times is a sign that there is an accepting intimacy between two significant others.

Finally, excrement is a symbolic representation of death that we ourselves produce and that, indeed, we cannot help producing in the very process of maintaining our lives. Perhaps it is for making death so intimate that we find excrement so repulsive (Frankfurt, 2005, p. 44–45). As I already mentioned, as Douglas noted, reflection on excrement suggests not only the dynamic relation of order to disorder, form to formlessness, but also being to nonbeing, and life to death (Douglas, 1966, p. 7).

Thus, from a psychoanalytic point of view, excrement is an unremarkable substance that can become a symbol of aggressive wishes: it can become for example, "a mortal insult, a representation of class struggle, or a desperate protest" (Praeger, 2007, p. 135), but probably most of all, it is meant to hurt the other in some kind of deeply personal manner which makes it eminently suitable for expressing justified or unjustified aggression at the target. As Haslam (2012) notes, scatological language has diverse purposes, it has at least three functions: it can be a way of expressing emotions, it is a form of communication meant to influence others and it is a way of self-regulating as in pain control in child birth.

Telephone Scatologia

Telephone scatologia is a paraphilic disorder (e.g., exhibitionism and voyeurism) such that sexual-erotic arousal and satisfaction are preconditioned upon talking about sexual or obscene topics (often of an anal nature) over the telephone to an anonymous listener. The term scatologia emanates from a Greek word *"skato"* for "dung" and logos for "speech," telephone scatologia can be literally translated as "dirty talking through the telephone." Telephone scatologia is a type of paraphilia categorized as "Other Specified Paraphilic Disorder" in Diagnostic and Statistical Manual-5 (Siddiqui et al., 2017).

Researchers have claimed that the typical "dirty" caller is a heterosexual man of average or raised sex drive, with no serious cognitive deficits and a history of failed relationships and/or truncated social interactions. Moreover, research suggests that there are three common types of callers: the first type is profane and immediately suggestive, the second lures the listener in and gradually leads them into offensive suggestions, and the third offender hoodwinks the listener into exposing personal information (Zidenberg & Won, 2015). Zidenberg and Won are mainly drawing from the important initial typology of obscene callers first articulated by Mead (1975).

As Griffiths (2017) summarizes the matter:

1   Type 1: These involve telephone callers who instantly curse and/or make obscene overtures, and are typically teenagers.
2   Type 2: These involve telephone callers described as "ingratiating seducers" that use a strategy (e.g., claiming they have mutual friends) before becoming more offensive.
3   Type 3: These involve telephone callers described as "tricksters" that use a subterfuge (e.g., pretending they are conducting a national survey) in order to discuss personal matters. This inevitably morphs into obscene and sexual overtures.

There are only a few theories as to how telephone scatophilia evolves (ibid). Kurt Freund, a deceased Czech-Canadian sexologist wrote numerous articles claiming that behaviors such as telephone scatophilia are generated by what he called *"courtship disorders"* (Freund & Blanchard, 1986). As Griffith's further notes, according to Freund, normal courtship includes four phases: (1) a finding phase, i.e., location and evaluation of a partner, (2) an affiliative phase, i.e., nonverbal and verbal pre-tactile interactions like looking, smiling and talking, (3) a tactile interaction phase in which physical contact is implemented and (4) genital union phase in which sexual intercourse occurs. Freund suggested that obscene telephone calling (and exhibitionism) is a disturbance of the second phase of the courtship disorder (Griffiths, 2017). Similarly, says Griffiths, Money (1986) proposed the *"lovemap"* theory suggesting that paraphiliac behavior happens when an abnormal lovemap develops which impedes and truncates the ability to engage in loving sexual intercourse. A lovemap is "a developmental representation or template in the mind and in the brain depicting the idealized lover and the idealized program of sexual and erotic activity projected in imagery or actually engaged in with that lover" (Money, 1986, p. 290). In this model, says Griffiths, "telephone scatologia, is classified as an allurement paraphilia involving the preparatory or courtship phase prior to genital intercourse" (Griffiths, 2017). While both of these models describe many cases of telephone scatophilia, there is some empirical evidence that some obscene telephone callers have courtship behavior that is within normal limits, which points to the ambiguity associated with this condition and its causation (ibid).

From a psychoanalytic point of view, what makes telephone scatologia an anal event is the way the caller relates to the victim, what Grunberger (1979) calls the "anal object." That is,

> what constitutes the essential character of the anal object relation is that the power ratio takes precedence over the very impulse that it would seem to have to underlie, by conveying the energy necessary for its gratification.... The energy basis of anal object relations is the control of the object and a certain *balance of power* that guarantees it.
>
> (Grunberger, 1979, p. 151)

As Freud implied the anal-sadistic phone caller prepares his victim by attacking him in order to be able to metaphorically devour him later (ibid. p. 155). Put in non-instinctual/energic terms, what the dirty phone caller wishes to do to his victim, regardless of his way of engaging the victim in terms of courtship disorders or lovemaps, is to make her into excrement, an anonymous mass of undifferentiated nothingness. That is, to assault her autonomy, integration and humanity—her dignity. Dirty callers are trying to rob the woman (typically) of all her dignity as a unique other, and to reduce her into a repository of his anal sadism: their rage at women, often beginning with their non-nurturing and non-stable mother, is aimed at reducing the woman into a toilet that they defecate into and onto. Obscene excretion and sexual language is the way this is usually implemented. This was certainly the case with my one patient who before the internet era (which has made toilet cursing and graffiti easier, including to reach more people), would from time to time call up anonymous women and say degrading words to her, often using excremental as well as sexual terms, including his wishes to perform anal sex, concluding in him masturbating to

the woman's negative reaction (during or after the call). What ultimately pleasured him he told me, was the squirming woman who was
ambushed by his telephonic intrusion (regardless of whether it was
Meade's Type 1, 2 or 3 approach). Needless to say, telephone scatalogia has its voyeuristic and exhibitionistic elements to it. What is
important for our discussion is that those who engage in telephone
scatologia are engaged in a deviant activity that is metaphorically and
practically a form of dung or excremental speech through the phone,
implicating the anal phase, anality and the like as a "go to" resource
to express violent emotion, usually hostile emotion directed at women
by men.[6]

Caprolalia

Caprolalia is the involuntary and repetitive use of obscene language,
as a symptom of mental illness or organic brain disease. Coprolalia
comes from the Greek *kópros*, meaning "dung, feces," and *laliã*
meaning "speech", from the verb to "to talk". Caprolalia is most
associated with vocal tics accompanying those suffering from Gilles de
al Tourettes syndrome. Most often these vocal tics are not said within
normative social or emotional contexts, and typically are spoken or
repeated compulsively in a louder tone or different cadence or pitch
than normative conversational speech. Especially embarrassing for
some individuals with coprolalia are involuntary outbursts within
social contexts, such as racial or ethnic slurs in the company of the
very people who would be most offended by such remarks. A minority
of people with coprolalia have this particular problem. It is crucial to
understand that these incendiary words or complex phrases do not
necessarily reflect the thoughts, beliefs or opinions of the person with
coprolalia. Some phrases can be quite complicated, often meaningless
and even amusing if not comical, which can be the butt of comedians
and others.

Psychoanalytically, at least historically, vocal tics were viewed as
psychologically motivated, though with regards to those vocal tics
associated with Tourette's syndrome, the evidence indicates that these
tics are genetically and neurologically caused and best treated with
medications. However, early analysts, including Freud viewed vocal
tics as related to hysterical symptoms, reflecting repressed sexual
(including masturbatory) and aggressive wishes, a perspective that has
largely been discredited when it comes to Tourette's syndrome. What is
psychoanalytically interesting is that the syndrome may occur in some
instances within the context of the totality of circumstances that the

person is in, thus reflecting their life experience in real time. In other words, caprolalia is not psychologically motivated, but it is psychologically informative and enlightening (Haslam, 2012). Indeed, the one Tourette's adolescent I treated many years ago was prone to scream and shout excremental and sexual terms, "shit head" and "fuck you" in contexts that were embarrassing such as when I went outside with him to get say a slice of pizza. Even though I discussed with him the social circumstances where we were going which was a treat for him as he told me, and that I wanted him to try and control his impulses to say outrageous things out loud (and he agreed to this), he most often succumbed to his impulsivity. In the transference I could not help feel that this lad had more control over his behavior than he displayed, and that part of his outburst were psychologically motivated, meant to embarrass me, which it did. When we returned to my office, and we discussed the happening, the patient smirked and appeared to be pleased that he put me in a socially compromised situation. Eventually, and with the right medication which I arranged with one of the Tourette's medical specialists, this kind of behavior was greatly lessoned, though not eliminated, suggesting that there was an interaction between biology and psychology in terms of his public outbursts with me. Many years later I ran into the patient and his Tourette's symptoms were curtailed though he had some episodic facial tics.

What the aforementioned discussion discloses is something that we all feel from time to time, namely, the wish to blurt something out that is radically inappropriate to the emotional and social context, for example, the impulse to shout excremental/sexual obscenities at a funeral. While most of the time we do not scream excremental/sexual obscenities at a funeral or at similarly serious and somber contexts (e.g., a religious mass), most of the time the reason behind wanting to scream for no obvious reason is frustration, anger, even hatred or some other form of ill-feeling toward the deceased. And not being able to express this negativity out on a person or situation is what causes the wish to just "let it out" in the form of screaming or yelling. Such screaming or yelling has an obsessive-compulsive "feel" to it, and calls to mind the anxiety that people feel when they want to act on an impulse that they know is not appropriate to the emotional and social context and may in fact generate guilt and/or shame. Many individuals with OCD report that these urges are undesired, but others get muddled because they worry that the reason the thoughts keep occurring is because they secretly want to act on them, which as an analyst, I believe is often the case. In other words, it is not simply there is a glitch in the inhibitory system, but an anti-social wish associated with the target person or situation. In the case of the funeral, my patient felt that the deceased was an awful husband, father and corrupt businessman who was being eulogized by the clergy and others as if he were a saint, and his wish to reveal the truth to the audience what a "low life" he was became almost impossible to contain. Instead of saying something out loud however, he engaged in private caprolalia (or caprolalia-like behavior), and gossiped to some of his friends who saw things likewise.

Caprophagia

Caprophagia is different than the caprologia associated with Tourette's syndrome which involves shouting excremental/sexual obscenities and other taboo words like *nigger* or *cunt* (the two of the most disgusting words in the English language by most accounts (Mohr, 2013, p. 9)). In coprophagia, we are dealing with the actual eating of excrement. The word is derived from the Greek *copros*, "feces" and *phagein*, "to eat". Coprophagy refers to many kinds of feces-eating, including eating feces of other species (heterospecifics), of other individuals (allocoprophagy), or one's own (autocoprophagy)—those once deposited or taken directly from the anus (Hirakawa, 2001).[7] It should be noted humans have no innate dislike to excrement and only come to acquire a disgust in early childhood. Children younger than 3, for example, show positive responses to fecal odours and in one study a majority of 2-year-olds put imitation dog feces in their mouths when it was offered to them on a plate (Rozin & Fallon, 1987, as cited in Haslam, 2012). In fact, consuming feces is minimally toxic. However, feces naturally include the bacteria typically found in the intestines. While these bacteria don't harm you when they're in your intestines, they are not healthy to be consumed in your mouth. Haslam (2012) aptly summarizes the varied meanings of coprophagia. Eating excrement, says Haslam, can serve diverse functions, it can illuminate many disorders, and be a manifestation of a variety of cognitions and wishes:

> It can be a compensation for lack of interpersonal connection, a regression to infantile modes of oral incorporation, a source of gustatory pleasure, a sign of disinhibition, an act of submission to powerful but imaginary figures, a form of penance, a desperate attempt to be clean, a sexual turn-on, or a symbol of madness.
> (Haslam, 2012, p. 113)

In psychoanalytic theory, coprophagia, has been viewed as a person's effort to reconstitute an insecure narcissistic balance, most often motivated by early loss of emotionally significant others. The "childhood loneliness" that is its consequence "is compensated by narcissistic over-valuation of bodily products", like fecal matter, "and by the symbolic reintrojection of what has been lost"(Akhtar, 2009, pp. 58–59; Tarachow, 1966).

Rather than go into the weird world of the extremely small minority of people who engage in coprophagia for sadomasochistic pleasure or as a consequence of extreme psychiatric or neurological conditions in our society, I wish to make one point that has bearing on those individuals who in their everyday lives are forced to "eat shit" or "eat shit and die," metaphorically speaking. As O'Neil (2018, n.p.) summarizes the matter, to tell a person to eat shit is to discharge them as undeserving of "the human-to-human response among equals that anything more elaborate implies." Aristophanes, says O'Neil, had a cheeky slave calling Asclepius a *skatophagus* (a shit eater) in Plutus all in about 380 B.C. To be an eater of shit is to be like a lowly animal. Dogs, continues O'Neil, consume their own excrement. Flies and dung beetles consume the excrement of other animals. Moreover, there is additionally an analogous sense of the meaning of the term eat shit. When skateboarders or snowboarders or athletes in other similar sports fall, says O'Neil, they say they ate shit, that is, they failed miserably. It is a common phrase to implore someone to eat your excrement, typically because they stole something from you (e.g., a sport victory). Eat shit is another way of saying "fuck you," but it is even more impersonal (ibid).

A Word on the Social Context of Cursing

Cursing is different in different cultures and conveys what the culture's main valuative attachments are (e.g., it has been alleged that Germans have a preference for abusive anal terms, based on their preoccupation with cleanliness (Haslam (2012)). Indeed, as Mohr (2013) points out in her brief history of cursing, *Holy Sh*t*, cursing provides a captivating record of what people care about on the profoundest levels of a culture, such as what is viewed as divine, what is regarded as terrifying, and what is judged as taboo. Other studies have supported Mohr's claims (Van Oudenhoven et al., 2008). However, it was Pinker (2007) who plausibly identified five likely purposes of cursing, which for our concerns is focused on excremental/urination themes. These examples are from college-age patients I have treated.

First, there is "abusive" cursing, which is meant to offend or intimidate and bring about psychological harm. For example, "you are a fucken asshole." Second, there is "cathartic cursing," which is implemented in situations of pain and misfortune. For example, "I can't take this leg pain shit anymore." Third, there is "dysphemistic" cursing, which is implemented to suggest that the speaker regards the topic under discussion in an unfavorable manner and wants the listener to feel likewise.[8] For example, "This god-damn calculus shit is irrelevant to my life." Fourth, "emphatic" cursing is meant to put into sharp focus what is judged by the speaker as worth attending to. "This Socratic dialogue crap is actually amazing to read." "Idiomatic" cursing, is implemented solely to show the speaker and listener are engaged in informal discussion. For example, "I really like that guy's ass, don't you?" Mohr has aptly summarized the numerous functions of cursing. She says that swearwords

> do what no other English words can. They are the most powerful words we have with which to express extreme emotion, whether negative or positive. They insult and offend others (which, like it or not, is a function of language); they offer catharsis as a response to pain or to powerful feelings; they cement ties among members of groups in ways that other words cannot.... We need irreproachable formal and unassailably decent speech, but we also need the dirty, the vulgar, the wonderful obscenities and oaths that can do for us what no other words can.
>
> (Mohr, 2013, pp. 14, 15)

What can psychoanalysis add to illuminating the motivations for toilet cursing in its extreme manifestation? After all, as Freud noted, psychoanalysis can be a useful tool for assisting us to comprehend what he called the "riddles of the world in which we live" (Freud, 1927, p. 253), "a key to the explanation of human phenomena in general (and not only pathological symptoms)" as Chasseguet-Smirgel (1984, p. 120) emphasized.

Perhaps there is no such place where the aggressive nature of toilet cursing occurs as in scatological humor. Comics have appropriated the extreme negativity of excrement to communicate in jokes and insults. It has unequivocal power to taint anything. But does scatological humor suggest something more about the human condition? Toilet humour is popular among a wide range of ages, but is especially popular with children and young teenagers, for whom cultural taboos related to acknowledgement of waste excretion still have a degree of amusing novelty. The humour comes from the rejection of such taboos, and is a part of modern culture. Examples can also be found in earlier literature, including *The Canterbury Tales* by Geoffrey Chaucer. As Evans further notes,

In English literature, scatological humour can be juvenile, but it has also been used to represent wider social anxieties. In turning bottoms up and exposing the rear end, "shiterature" is often about breaking taboos, and exposing the dirty underbelly of society. Part of the "civilising" process that societies perform to reach a high level of sophistication involves distancing oneself from one's own excrement, and scatology reverses this by shedding a light on our dirtiest natural habits. Swift's excremental vision asked us to peel back the mask of genteel individuals, revealing their true and disgusting selves.

(Evans, 2021, n.p.)

Some Clinical Implications of Toilet Cursing

Within the clinical context cursing (including toilet cursing) has a role that is often underappreciated in that it opens up domains of relating that are often overlooked, and of which cursing is a most direct and evocative way of conveying an insight to an analysand. In this section I want to give three simple examples of how cursing can have a positive impact on the treatment process, especially with people who regard cursing as part of how they reside in the world. Toilet cursing can serve several distinct and potentially valuable functions in treatment.

Of course, I am not saying, let alone advocating that toilet cursing, or cursing in general is a particularly "high level" sublimation of aggression or the like, but in some contexts, it can be a positive outlet for self-expression and creativity. For instance, some have claimed (Byrne, 2017) that cursing can stimulate very creative words as they curse, or they generate the motivation to complete an assignment or a project that has been disregarded or abandoned for many months or longer. In fact, cursing is a formidable shortcut, an emotionally infused aspect of language that allows us to communicate complex notions in a pressing manner. One patient of mine told me that learning how to curse in a skillful manner actually "liberated me" in other areas of his life. Cursing, says Byrne, including excremental cursing can help a person endure pain, work collectively, and communicate strong emotions.

Certain toilet curse words epitomize the concept of "economy of words." There are impressively few words that have the ability to communicate a notion and raw emotion in a single syllable. Shit (and fuck) are lodged in this select category. For example, a patient of mine told me "I don't give a shit what my boss thinks," an expression that makes it abundantly clear how angry, actually oppositional and defiant my patient felt. I responded that "for someone who does not 'give a shit' about your boss you seem to be rather explosively angry, like you would like to shit all over him." He concurred, as both the patient and I used the toilet curse word as shorthand in that it gave color and emphasis to the point being made. It also enhanced our social/emotional connection.

With a second patient who had a tendency to see things in black and white, in all or nothing terms, the word shit was used somewhat differently than the above example. For instance, this patient was prone to perfectionism and when his behavior was not up to snuff, such as not getting the highest grade in his law school class, he felt terrible about himself. That is, the word shit was used as a marker for his radically reduced self-esteem at not being the best in his class. He could not reside in the world of half-tints and gray, if he found himself on the wrong side of the bifurcation of good or bad, he regarded himself as a "shit head" as he called himself. As Stephen King noted somewhere, "oh shit it's shit."

A third patient was a control freak who could not tolerate the fact that things happen that are out of his control. Once, when he felt that he was the dominant one in a conversation, the other person reversed the course of the discussion leaving my patient feeling defeated. As he told me, and I agreed, citing the famous quote "people change, shit happens, life goes on." With this patient and the other two above, it was the working through of the meaning of the word shit that was pivotal in moving the analysis forward.

Conclusion: Redemption through the Carnivalesque

Despite most of us being raised to believe that all cursing is an absolute "no no" in terms of respectable presentation of the self in everyday life, cursing has a well-documented positive side. As Mark Twain famously noted in one of his many comments on the benefits of cursing, "The idea that no gentleman ever swears is all wrong. He can swear and still be a gentleman if he does it in a nice and benevolent and affectionate way." Moreover, "profanity provides a relief denied even to prayer" (www.twainquotes.com, profanity retrieved 2/8/21). As I already mentioned, in her provocative book Emma Byrne (2017) examined cutting-edge research to how cursing, at least in certain contexts can be psychologically and socially beneficial. Not only have some forms of cursing been in play since the earliest humans learned to communicate, but they have been demonstrated to diminish physical pain, to decrease anxiety, to prevent physical violence, to assist trauma victims reclaim language, and to facilitate human trust and cooperation in the workplace and at home. Cursing can express "anger, surprise, dismay, pain and disappointment, fear and sudden unhappiness," among other strong emotions (Haslam, 2012, p. 94). Toilet cursing, is a particular subspecies of the psychology of cursing, and when it is skillfully employed say in a humorous context, by a stand-up comic, an amateur, or even to oneself in a non-humorous manner, it can facilitate some positive psychological developments that help a person to press on amidst his trial and tribulations say at work or at home, and maybe even help fashion a flourishing life.[9]

It was the Russian philosopher Mikhail Bakhtin who has given us a clue on how one can look at excretion that rejects fecal denial and makes the "lower body stratum" (e.g. eating, drinking and defecating) as he called it, less objectionable as it is usually viewed. Bakhtin explored the laughter, parody and "grotesque realism" as he described it in his famous study of the medieval carnival. Bakhtin summarizes the main thrust of this study:

It could be said (with certain reservations, of course) that a person of the Middle Ages lived, as it were, *two lives*: one that was the *official* life, monolithically serious and gloomy, subjugated to a strict hierarchical order, full of terror, dogmatism, reverence and piety; the other was the *life of the carnival square*, free and unrestricted, full of ambivalent laughter, blasphemy, the profanation of everything sacred, full of debasing and obscenities, familiar contact with everyone and everything. Both these lives were legitimate, but separated by strict temporal boundaries.

(Brandist, 2021, n.p.)

The activities of the carnival square, says Brandist, collective criticism of officialdom, "inversion of hierarchy, violations of decorum and proportion, celebration of bodily excess and so on" express for Bakhtin, "an implicit popular conception of the world.... The carnivalesque becomes a set of image-borne strategies" for deconstructing the official worldview (ibid).

What Bakhtin was advocating in his study of the medieval carnival was a "liberating laughter," a freeing from the repression of the lower bodily stratum. He in effect turned excrement into something positive and good, it was the carnivalesque, a form of "scatological redemption" (Praeger, 2007 p. 200). As Praeger further noted,

> it is something you want to be contaminated with.... No longer the most extreme negative, it is the most extreme redemption. Carnivalesque laughter is not mocking, but inclusive, in that it exposes the impossibility of the ideals the voice of civilization mandates.
>
> (ibid, p. 201)

Carnivalesque laughter recognizes this untruth—you acknowledge that your body is defective, and you acknowledge that all bodies are defective, "and you realize that this doesn't make all humanity equally bad," rather "this makes all humanity equally good" (ibid.). Bakhtin identified this as the "material bodily principle," it is the comprehension that we all respond to a lower power, it is in fact, a rejection of "shameful shitting" (ibid). Moreover, says Praeger, the possibility for the carnivalesque exists in each culture. Such a portrayal of excrement, the contemporary carnivalesque—"that which threatens the Victorian legacy of fecal denial that drives our views of bodily functions and the epidemic of shameful shitting" (ibid.) This amounts to a positive characterization of excrement. The carnivalesque is a remarkable and "wonderful vision" (ibid., p. 203). Skillful, lighthearted toilet cursing as Mark Twain described it, is a form of the carnivalesque and their lies its positivity.

Notes

1 Scatolgical language is sometimes amalgamated with obscenity, vulgarity and slurs (Haslam, 2012).
2 I have drawn from Haslam (2012) who has used these three scatological examples in his chapter on "potty mouth."
3 Brown (1991) noted that, in his article "The Ontogenesis of the Interest in Money" Sandor Ferenczi had his intriguing conclusion, "After what has been said money is seen to be nothing other than deodorized, dehydrated shit that has been made to shine" (p. 179). Transforming feces to gold. However, it was Freud who first made the link between anality and money (Freud, 1908, pp. 173–174).
4 Haslam (2012) in his excellent review of the literature on the anal character or personality concludes that there is evidence in support of the coherence of anal traits; moreover, there is evidence that there is something truly anal about the anal character; however, there is no compelling evidence that the origin of the anal character is in toilet training.

5   As Praeger (2007, p. 126) notes, David Inglis (2001) claims that excremental insults fall into two groups: devaluing someone by linking him with the physical aspects of excrement (e.g., how the crowd insulted Jesus at his crucifixion), or defining someone by the manner in which he defecates e.g., (not using flush toilets when they first came out, or the public defecating in say India).

6   There is much less of this kind of behavior among women towards men cited in the literature.

7   Feces-eating has been connected to pica in childhood. Pica is defined as the propensity to eat substances that are not normally eaten, such as chalk, ashes, hair, paper and even feces, often looking like an obsessive-compulsive disorder (Haslam, 2012).

8   Pinker does not include dysphemistic cursing in his list of "five ways to cuss." Rather he uses the category he calls "'descriptively,' (*Let's fuck*)'" However, he discusses dysphemistic as follows: "The major difference is that the taboo terms is dysphemistic—it calls to mind the most disagreeable aspects of the referent, rather than just pointing to it" (Pinker, 2007, p. 350).

9   Bathroom humor typically involves coarse references to bodily functions like defecating, urinating and vomiting. I am not in general, advocating resorting to coarse bathroom humor for self-enhancement, though sometimes such bathroom-like humor has its place when it is implemented in a lighthearted or other potentiating manner. It is worth noting that researchers have not come up with any agreed upon typical cursing personality or psychiatric diagnostic category, though there have been some lose associations say between anti-social types and cursing and depression in adolescence (Haslam, 2012). Men tend to curse more than women, and each gender tends to view it differently and they are targeted differently. For example, Haslam notes that "women are more often targets of taboo animal terms (e.g., bitch), revealing a deeper, lingering connection between women and beasts" (Haslam, 2012, p. 100).

References

Abraham, K. (1924). *The influence of oral eroticisms on character formation. In: Selected Papers of Karl Abraham, M.D.* New York: Brunner-Mazel, 393–406.

Akhtar, S. (2009). *Comprehensive Dictionary of Psychoanalysis.* London: Karnac.

Chasseguet-Smirgel, J. (1985). *Creativity and Perversion.* New York: W.W. Norton & Company.

Brandist, C. (2021). Bakhtin Circle. *The Internet Encyclopedia*, n.p., retrieved April 26, 2022.

Brown, N.O. (1991). *Apocalypse and/or Metamorphosis.* Berkeley: University California Press.

Byrne, E. (2017). *Swearing Is Good For You. The Amazing Science Of Bad Language.* New York: W.W. Norton & Company.

Douglas, M. (1966). *Purity and Danger. An analysis of concept of pollution and taboo.* London: Routledge.

Evans, P. (2021) Poo jokes and pessimism – the scatological legacy of British humour Is it simply a testament to our good nature, or a sign of a darker kind of cynicism? *The New Statesman*, UK Edition. https://www.newsta tesman.com, retrieved January 11, 2022.

Frankfurt, H.G. (2005). *On Bullshit*. Princeton: Princeton University Press.

Freud, S. (1908). Character and anal eroticism. In *The Standard Edition of the Complete Psychological Works of Sigmund Freud*, Trans J. Strachey with A. Freud assisted by A. Stratchey and A. Tyson, 24 volumes (1953–1974). London: Hogarth Press and the Institute of Psycho-Analysis, vol. 9, 167–175. (Henceforth *S.E.*)

Freud, S. (1913). Foreword. In J.G. Bourke [1891]. *The Portable Scatalog. Excerpts from Scatological Rites of All Nations. A Dissertation upon the Employment of Excrementations Remedial Agents in Religion, Therapeutics, Divination, Witchcraft, Love-Philters, etc., in all Parts of the Globe.* Edited by L.P. Kaplan. New York: William Morrow and Company, 5–9.

Freud, S. (1917). Post-script to a Discussion on Lay Analysis. S.E., 20, 251–258.

Freud, S. (1918). From the History of Infantile Neurosis. S.E., 17, 1–122.

Freud, S. (1927). Post-script to a Discussion of Lay Analysis. S.E. 20, 251–258.

Freund, K. and Blanchard, R. (1986). The concept of courtship disorder. *Journal of Sex & Marital Therapy*, 12, 79–92.

Gregory, M.E. and James, S. (2009). *Toilets of the World*. London: Merrell.

Griffiths, M.D. (2017). The Psychology of Obscene Telephone Calling. A Brief look at telephone scatologia. https://www.psychologytoday.com, retrieved February 2, 2017.

Grunberger, B. (1979). *Narcissism. Psychoanalytic Essays*. New York: International Universities Press.

Haslam, N. (2012). *Psychology in the Bathroom*. New York: Palgrave Macmillan.

Hirakawa, H (2001). Coprophagy in leporids and other mammalian herbivores." *Mammal Review*, 31 (1), 61–80.

Inglis, D. (2001) *A Sociological History of Excretory Experience: Defecatory Manners and Toiletry Technologies*. New York: Edwin Mellen Press.

Mead, B.T. (1975). Coping with obscene phone calls. *Medical Aspects of Human Sexuality*, 9, 127–128.

Mohr, M. (2013). *Holy Shit. A Brief history of Swearing*. Oxford: Oxford University Press.

Money, J. (1986). *Lovemaps: Clinical Concepts of Sexual/Erotic Health and Pathology, Paraphilia, and Gender Transposition in Childhood, Adolescence, and Maturity.* New York: Prometheus Books.

O'Neil, L. (2018). "Eat Shit" is The Singular Insult of These Profoundly Stupid Times. *Esquire*. https://www.esquire.com, retrieved April 26, 2022.

Pinker, S. (2007). *The Stuff of Thought*. New York: Viking.

Praeger, D. (2007). *Poop Culture. How America is Shaped By Its Grossest National Product.* Los Angeles: Ferral House.

Rozin, P. & Fallon, A. (1987). A perspective on disgust. *Psychological Review*, 94, 23–41.

Shengold, L. (1988). *Hale In The Sky. Observations On Anality And Defense.* New Haven: Yale University Press.

Siddiqui, J.A., Qureshi, S.F. & A. Al Zahrani, A. (2017). Verbal Exhibitionism: A Brief Synopsis of Telephone Scatologia. *Indian Journal of Mental Health,* 4 (2), 109–114.

Tarachow, S. (1966). Coprohagia and Allied Phenomena *Journal of the American Psychoanalytic Association,* 14: 685–699.

Van Oudenhoven, J.P., de Raad, B., Askevis-Lehherpeux, E., Boski, P., Brunborg, G.S., Carmona, C., Barelds, D., Hill, C.T., Mlačić, B., Motti, F., Rammsteadt, B., and Woods, S. (2008). Terms of abuse as expression and reinforcement of cultures. *International Journal of Intercultural Relations,* 32, 174–185.

Wiseman, J (1996). *SM101. A Realistic Introduction.* 2nd edition. San Francisco: Greenery Press.

Zidenberg, A.M. & Won, P. (2015). Telephone Scatologia. A Review of the Literature. *Inquiries. Social Sciences, Arts, and Humanities,* 7 (9), 1–9.

Chapter 5

Public Bathroom Graffiti

Bathroom wall graffiti (henceforth, graffiti) refers to marks, scratchings or drawings usually made on the walls of the stall where one defecates (though it can be on other parts of the bathroom, like the urinal). It has a long history that goes back to the ancient Romans and Greeks. In this chapter, I want to review what we know about scatological graffiti, though most graffiti is a creative combination of themes such as "scatological political insults, sexual humour, self-referential hostility" and unclassifiable graffiti that reflects the idiosyncratic trajectory of the person drawing the graffiti (Haslam, 2012, p. 120). It is worth noting that there is no single personality type that engages in bathroom wall graffiti, thus the reasons why one does so are varied. My claim is that the main thrust of such graffiti is that it is a form of storytelling, an artistic expression and play that has the unique feature of being anonymously written and anonymously read. By virtue of being anonymous from both ends as it were, a person who creates graffiti can be truthful, and the reader also especially enjoys the brute honesty of the marks, scratchings or drawings. This is an important observation, that those who create bathroom graffiti only receive anonymous recognition and no financial benefit. As one graffiti author wrote tongue and cheek, "Since writing on the toilet walls is neither for critical acclaim, nor financial rewards, it is the purest form of art – Discuss" (www.boredpanda.com/inspirational-bathroom-stall, retrieved January 20, 2022).

Psychoanalytic Speculations on Graffiti

Gadpaille (1974) viewed graffiti as a self-administered living Rorschach of individuals in society.[1] In this view, graffiti is something of a failsafe for unconscious forbidden wishes and thoughts and is mainly a way of aggressively violating social prohibitions by defying social

DOI: 10.4324/9781003219705-5

taboos. In other words, there is a link between defecation and the aggressive nature of wall writing. Other speculations include the usual suspects of psychoanalytic theorizing: for men graffiti is a phallic striving, such that the pen is symbolically equivalent to the penis as a vehicle for self-assertion, to make a mark on the world (Landy & Steele, 1967); some heterosexual men draw male anatomy and sexual function as an unconscious manifestation of their homosexual wishes and desires (Kinsey et al., 1953). In this view, since all graffiti is usually meant for a same sex audience, there is something intrinsically homosexual about graffiti (the same may be for women in our era); graffiti is an aggressive expression on the bathroom wall itself. Walls epitomize our separation from others and calls to mind our remoteness from others.[2] Lomas also equates graffiti to understanding dreams, jokes, and slips of the tongue, and like these behaviors, it is the relation of the writer to the wall that holds the master key to understanding graffiti (Lomas, 1973, 1976, 1980). As Lomas notes,

> The use of the wall for drawing pictures or making jokes is to point out that the wall itself is no joke, and no art gallery, and no artistic creating, but rather a necessity to keep the inside in and outside out.
>
> (Lomas, 2013, p. 83)

Haslam summarizes this point, "toilet graffiti are therefore a form of aggressive protest against the wall for what it represents and a kind of exhibitionistic hostility towards the captive audience that is forced to view it" (Haslam, 2012, p. 132). Moreover, the blank wall is like an empty screen in which we project our ungratified wishes, including reading the scribblings on the walls, that frequently reflect childlike "polymorphous perverse behavior" (i.e., infantile sexuality) (Lomas, 1973, p. 80). Finally, Dundes (1966) who invented the term latrinalia suggests that there is a uniquely anal erotic aspect to latrinalia that is analogous to fecal smearing. Dirty words on bathroom walls are symbolically analogous to excrement and by writing them people are discharging the childish impulses towards bodily filth that are typically later sublimated in adulthood (Haslam, 2012, p. 133). Drawing from Bettelheim's *Symbolic Wounds*, Dundes further claims that this anal dynamic may help to illuminate what he believes is men's greater inclination to write graffiti (however, in our age, men and women probably engage in graffiti about equally). Men unconsciously envy women their ability to give birth, and regard defecation as a substitute. Women, not needing such an alternative, are less in need of what Dundes calls "faecal substitute activities" such as bathroom wall graffiti, sculpture, painting, and blowing wind instruments (ibid). Dunde's provocative theory says Haslam, does not adequately account for the fact that women, like men, engage in considerable bathroom graffiti.

There is little doubt that there is plausibility to the aforementioned speculations about what may be motivating a particular person to engage in graffiti at a particular time, though some of the speculations appear to be dated if not unconvincing. In truth one would have to have a particular person on the couch as it were to explore the meaning of his graffiti and even then, one never knows for sure if one has put the main motivation into sharp focus. This being said, I would like to offer a complimentary point of view about graffiti, namely, it is a form of storytelling, the shortest of short stories, it is a barely sublimated form of artistic expression and it is a form of play. Before doing so however, I want to say a brief word about the social psychological and sociological explanations of bathroom graffiti.

Latranalia can be viewed as a manifestation of "dominant social values" (Haslam, 2012, p. 133). For example, says Haslam, the fact that there is less prevalence of homosexual graffiti in say the Philippines compared to the U.S. is probably because there is greater acceptance of graffiti in the U.S. Likewise, the fact that there is less solicitation of homosexual graffiti in the U.S. compared to earlier times is probably because there has been a liberalizing of social values and attitudes. As Haslam notes, there are "parallels between cultural preoccupations of a group and the themes of its wall scratching" (ibid.). Latranalia has also been viewed as a "societal symptom" (ibid., p. 134). That is, graffiti has been explained as not a reflection of society's dominant values, but a form of protest against them. In this view, "when some values become dominant it leads people to express their opposition to these values in covert and underground ways," such as bathroom graffiti (ibid.). For example, says Haslam, "homophobic graffiti may increase as social attitudes become less anti-gay and racist graffiti may be more prevalent in liberal academic settings, where expression of racist sentiments is less acceptable, than in other public settings" (ibid.). Thus, bathroom wall graffiti does not simply reflect dominant values, but are a reaction and rebellion against these values as the "symptomatic expression of hidden conflict and dissent" (ibid.).

Graffiti as Storytelling

The story telling experience of the reader of graffiti have their unique context-dependent, setting-specific rhythms of perception and emotion, what they have in common with other forms of storytelling is the power to galvanize, to stimulate great internal activity that feels not only uplifting, but also transformative, at least to some degree to the reader (and the author).[3] The fact that such graffiti has been called "shithouse poetry" or the "poetry of the smallest room" speaks to this point (Dundes, 1966, p. 91). As Lomas notes in another context, "there is something magical about writing on bathroom walls" (and reading them) (Lomas, 1973, p. 80). One graffiti author wrote poetry, "Here I sit broken-hearted, came to shit, but only farted. Later on I took my chance, came to fart but shit my pants," while another wrote "Ministry of Magic" above the toilet wall. A third example from a bathroom wall, "The chamber of secrets is in the next stall" (www. boredpanda.com/inspirational-bathroom-stall, retrieved January 20, 2022). That is, the reader of graffiti in his private experience of reading the bathroom wall can feel he has engaged in a positively transforma-tional dialogue, especially if he adds to the graffiti, whether literally or in phantasy. However, this is a dialogue with a fantasized phantom author and that is what makes such graffiti particularly interesting, as I said, the anonymity from both sides which invites truth-telling because the narcissistic investment in the graffiti is not operative in the same way as authored/named material is. In this view, often in an amusing manner, the reader is "reminded of some aspect of who they really are or would like to become, or forming some other connection with" these perspective-altering scratches, markings and drawings. It is as if the reader has "viewed an unnoticed window through which they have viewed some large or small piece of life" (Lippman, 1999, pp. 207–208).

Graffiti like all storytelling "is the commodity of all human beings, in all places, in all times. It is used to educate, inspire, to record his-torical events, to entertain and to transmit cultural mores" (Collins & Cooper, 2005, p. 1). This is the social aspect of graffiti, it relates to the values and problems in society which the author is trying to put right using the bathroom wall as his vehicle.

Compared to acting, where one has memorized lines to precisely say while remaining concentrated on the role and place in the story, in graffiti storytelling the author has greater freedom and power, for in his creations he has to "to make the light, sound, the action and all the character come alive," in a word or two, or a simple drawing (ibid., 61). Like other forms of storytelling, graffiti can define and demarcate relationships and generate parameters; they give a sense of self-coherence, self-continuity, and self-esteem, for they provide an account (at least a partial one) of who we are, where we came from and where we want to go, including conveying our most cherished values. In other words, these short stories are the repository for our most profound "longings, hopes, and fears"; such stories also interrogate life by encouraging critical self-reflection and "put[ing] up a mirror to yourself and to culture" (Harvey, 2012, p. 4). As Ferem noted whether public bathroom graffiti "is a knee-jerk reaction to our collective malaise or the process of our psychic healing, it wills itself into existence, and on some level this may be validation enough" (Ferem, 1964, p. 17). Finally, more than "facts," graffiti stories reveal "usable truths" as philosopher Richard Rorty called them, truths that convey meaning to our experiences and direction to our live (1989, pp. 4–6). In graffiti, the author is trying to evoke strong, well-placed emotion, for this is what makes the reader feel he is "included" in the story. One graffiti author wrote, "Be fearless – fart as loud as your anus will allow," while another wrote "Everyone hates a racist. But racists only hate a few people" (there is an accompanying picture of a sad face, www.boredpanda.com/inspirational-bathroom-stall, retrieved January 20, 2022). It is worth noting that storytellers need to find the right repertoire, as they see it, that is most in sync with their outlook on life and that uses emotions that the teller comfortably works with, even a few lines on a toilet wall. "The truth of art", including graffiti and all storytelling, said Constantin Stanislavski, "is the truth of your given circumstances." The "given circumstances" are the situations in which the actor finds himself during a play or in the case of the graffiti writer, his "storying" situation (Marcus & Marcus, 2011, p. 50). Perhaps the essence of graffiti is the ability to create new realities, to actualize what is unthinkable and unimaginable what is "not yet." When we see "great" graffiti, we feel there is something rather remarkable going on, as what is a normative aspect of experience, going to the toilet, has morphed into something appealingly otherwise, something new, thanks to the graffiti. One graffiti author wrote on a door stall, "Do you idealize the past or see it as broken? Why? While the reader responded, 'Dude. I'm just trying to take a shit'." (www.bor edpanda.com/inspirational-bathroom-stall, retrieved January 20, 2022).

It is via the author's "retellings" that we are able to see the material in question from a different slant, in a "new" way that gives new "reality" to, or puts into sharp focus what was previously not seen. In a sense the author's inner most self is being revealed, at least a bit of it, without deploying his usual defenses. This can be because he feels "close" to his imagined reader, or sufficiently distant to reveal important to him aspects of himself. One might say that the author of graffiti is playing with his imagined reader. To achieve this kind of openness to the reader requires a dimunition of one's narcissism, one's need for self-aggrandizement and the like. On the other hand, graffiti may reflect the opposite, the need for self-affirmation.

Two simple examples of graffiti, qua storytelling, were described to me by two different patients I treated many years ago. The first patient was going through a terrible breakup of a relationship with a woman that he loved but she wanted out of the relationship for no compelling reason (it sounded to me that she had grown out of him). He confided in me that he had written in a bathroom stall in Citi Field stadium the following: "Shiela is an asshole, she sucked my dick but won't give me the time of day now." In addition, he drew a picture of a woman on a horse riding into the sunset, never looking back, with my patient standing there with a sad face. My patient said that he felt a kind of relief depicting his experience and hoped that other men who were going through what he was would identify with it and feel they are not alone in their experience of being abandoned for no good reason as he put it. The patient felt a sense of uplifting relief after writing/drawing the graffiti. Needless to say, the theme of abandonment was played out in the transference as well, especially around vacations.

A second female patient wrote on the bathroom wall where she worked that "the bosses are assholes, they stink at what they do." She too drew a picture, of towering men whipping her and her fellow female workers, calling to mind the feeling of slavery to an authoritarian task master. My patient hated her job, and had wanted out for many years but felt trapped for a variety of financial and other reasons. She further told me that she felt she was getting back at those "asinine bosses," who "don't give a shit how they treat people, especially the women working in the corporation" (she sounded believable to me). When I asked her if she felt a bit guilty for defacing the bathroom wall which did not belong to her, she told me "not for a minute," that they deserved what was written because of their mistreatment of her, and the fact that she did not have any effective way of fighting back, hence the graffiti. Again, needless to say, my patient played out these dynamics at least to some extent, in the treatment with me, often seeing me as a "boss" man who wouldn't let her be herself.

In both of these vignettes we see the function of graffiti storytelling: it is a release valve to strong emotions that they believed they could not adequately express to the offending persons. In addition, both writers of the graffiti believed that their messages would be read by many likeminded people and would agree with them, hence giving them the feeling of being somewhat elevated via the graffiti.

Graffiti as Art

Graffiti can be viewed as a popular art form, including a way of social expression and communication (Lomas, 1976). Not only is it a cultural artifact but it can be conceptualized as a medium of expression (Ferem, 1964). Graffiti in the bathroom can reasonably be viewed as a form of Street Art. Street art is visual art created in public contexts for public viewing. It therefore requires a degree of creativity, creativity psychoanalytically defined as "the capacity to arrive at novel but valid solutions to problems... the capacity to create imaginative products which are compelling, convincing, significant etc." (Rycroft, 1995, p. 29). Graffiti is different from Street Art, for example, street art is typically painted with permission or it is commissioned while graffiti is technically vandalism.[4] Graffiti is word-based, whereas Street Art is typically image based. This being said, what exactly is artistic about graffiti written and drawn in the bathroom?

1   Graffiti is in sync with the common definition of art: The Oxford dictionary defines art as "the expression or application of human creative skill and imagination, typically in a visual form such as painting or sculpture, producing works to be appreciated primarily for their beauty or emotional power" (The Oxford Pocket Dictionary of Current English, 2000, online).
2   Whether image or word based, it is a form of self-expression and can transmit powerful ideas and messages that can influence people on a regular basis.
3   The creator of graffiti has to sublimate his wishes and desires in a manner that is often transparently animated by unconscious processes, especially infantile sexuality when it comes to the bathroom context, e.g., the anal phase of psychosexual development.
4   Graffiti tries to "arrive at novel but valid solutions to problems [at least to the author]... the capacity to create imaginative products which are compelling, convincing, significant etc." (at least to the author and reader) which is why it is regarded by some as captivating. The problems are those that the author finds summoning which often resonate with the reader.

While I have no intention of reviewing the various psychoanalytic formulations about what the artistic process is, my sense based on my clinical experience and what I have read is that the creation process used by the author of graffiti (and resonates with the reader), is aptly described by the Kleinian perspective. In this account, creativity is either depressive or schizoid, that is, it either represents an effort to make reparation for destructive fantasies, or is in some way analogous to the delusional system-making of schizophrenics (Rycroft, 1995). Indeed, as the afore-mentioned examples suggest, the author of graffiti is often trying to repair, or put right some perceived injury to his sense of self-coherence, self-continuity and self-esteem. The depressive position emphasizes that it is when the infant/patient/graffiti author(?) realizes that both his love and hate are directed at the same object, the main parental caregiver, and that he has ambivalence to the caregiver, that he attempts to shield the care-giver from his hatred by making reparations. Likewise, in the paranoid-schizoid phase, the infant/patient/graffiti author(?) copes with his innate destructive impulses by splitting both his ego and his object representa-tion into good and bad parts, and projecting his destructive impulses on to the bad object by who he feels persecuted (ibid., pp. 36, 125). In this way the graffiti author often presents his material in terms of good and bad, with very little half tints or the gray area. Whether referring to those people who have offended the author, or other forms of scatological like those that have a humorous motivation, we sense the depressive and paranoid processes may be in play. For example, "Our butt cheek have touched the same surface. We are one brothers. We are one."

And another, "Don't be a dick—Plato." And finally, "I think therefore I poop. I poop, therefore I am—Descartes"[5] (www.boredpanda.com/inspirational-bathroom-stall, retrieved 1/20/22).

Graffiti as Play

It is obvious that on some level those who create graffiti on the bathroom walls are having fun, just as the reader of graffiti is enjoying himself. That is, such graffiti is a form of play, especially when it incorporates bath-room humor. Indeed, there probably is a developmental pathway from children who play with their feces, including smearing them, to say playing with the modeling compound Play-Do, to finger painting, sand play etc., and finally to graffiti. This being said, graffiti is not exactly like children's play, though it is a "lower-level" form of sublimated activity. I say lower-level form because so much graffiti actually depicts themes of defecation, urination and the like. A whimsical example of graffiti:

> I love that girl with the little red shoes. She spends my money and drinks my booze. She don't have a cherry but that's not a sin cause she still has the box the cherry came in.
> (www.boredpanda.com/inspirational-bathroom-stall, retrieved 1/20/22)

It was Donald Winnicott who famously wrote about play in the most interesting manner, and some of his ideas have bearing in understanding graffiti as play. Briefly, Winnicott viewed playing as a developmental accomplishment, and situated it in the "intermediate area of experience" between the infant and the mother (the "third area," "potential space," and "transitional space"). Intermediate area of experience refers to the place where imagination emanates and paradox is amplified (paradox in the sense that some activities are real and unreal including at the same time). It is place where cultural experience occurs (Akhtar, 2009). As Akhtar further notes, it is "the space between (1) the subjectively perceived environment mother and objectively perceived object mother, (2) the child's experience of unity with and separateness from the mother, and (3) the ego's perception of reality and unreality" (ibid., p. 215). Moreover, for Winnicott "'play' was an imaginative elaboration of thoughts and feelings about the body, object relations and anxieties. Play enriches life, and enjoyment of playing is a hallmark of the growing child's mental health" (ibid., p. 211). For Winnicott, play emanated from the "deepest" part of the child (that which is inherited and orients the child, ultimately the "true self"), and involved being imaginative and original. The function of play for Winnicott, and the subsequent analysts was mainly striving for mastery over internal conflicts and external dangers, an ego-enhancing activity. Play typically evolves into more and more complex forms as the child gets older, that enhance the ego's effectiveness in managing the inner and outer worlds (ibid. p. 212).

In what way is scatological graffiti a form of play? First, it is clearly an imaginative elaboration of thoughts and feelings about the body, object relations and anxieties. Second, the goal of graffiti appears to be striving for some kind of mastery over internal conflicts and less but still, outer dangers. Thirdly, graffiti has a family resemblance to free association, in that the scratchings, marks and drawings seem to be spontaneous. They are not typically scripted as in play. Fourth, graffiti appears to be done for its own sake to gain pleasure, it does not have any serious aims and ends, in contrast to work (Rycroft, 1995) (in fact, analysts believe that the infant/child's "work" is to elaborate his play with the help of facilitating care givers). Fifth, the graffiti artist is at the same time expressing phantasy and accommodating to the external world, the latter at least to some degree (ibid.) (notwithstanding the fact the graffiti is technically vandalism, creation and destruction are its core). Sixth, like play, the author's individual solitary graffiti is engaged in a communal-like activity since the purpose of the graffiti is that it be read by an anonymous other. In other words, at least on the level of phantasy, it is sociable and inter-active. This is especially the case in those somewhat rare instances where a graffiti artist and his reader communicate with each other through the back-and-forth graffiti, calling to mind Winnicott's squiggle game. In the squiggle game, says Akhtar, the analyst draws a wave-like line or figure on a sheet of paper and asks the child/patient to add to it or to draw something of his own design, to which Winni-cott could further elaborate, if not detail. He and the child then took turns to finish some kind of a picture from their random-like draw-ings. Allegedly, the squiggle game, somewhat like graffiti, is like a dream, that expresses the unconscious of the child, though it could be therapeutic for its own sake (Akhtar, 2009, p. 270). Seventh, like play, graffiti usually eliminates any inhibitions or guilt in the author and therefore allows repressed wishes to emerge (Rycroft, 1995). Eighth, like play, graffiti is a form of communication. Ninth, like play, graffiti has an adventuresome and risky side to it in that it is a form of vandalism. Tenth, like play, graffiti is an active phenomenon, where spontaneity and surprise are emphasized. Eleventh, like play, certain forms of scatological graffiti are symbolic, though this is usually not the case.

While play is a huge topic in psychoanalytic thought, I have simply suggested some parallels between play in children and authoring sca-tological graffiti. Needless to say, this is a ripe subject for further investigation.

Conclusion

Scatological graffiti, like all types of bathroom graffiti can usefully be conceptualized as derivatives from the repressed, similar to dreams, jokes and slips of the tongue. That is, such graffiti whether viewed as storytelling, artistic expression or play, seems to centrally express anally-based and animated sexual and aggressive material. As with dreams, jokes and slips of the tongue, the person's associations are what matter most to get the best sense of what the graffiti sketching's, marks and pictures actually mean. This being said, in general those who write graffiti probably feel unnoticed and powerless in their everyday lives and therefore resort to graffiti to make their mark in this alienating if not hostile world. Graffiti in other words, is a beacon drawing our focus to a pervasive spiritual disconnect (Ferem, 1964). As the great street artist Bansky noted, "Graffiti is one of the few tools you have if you have almost nothing. And even if you don't come up with a picture to cure world poverty you can make someone smile while they're having a piss"[6] (https://quotes.thefamouspeople.com, banksy-669, retrieved 1/20/22).

Notes

1 I have liberally drawn from Haslam's (2012) succinct and thoughtful summary of the psychoanalytic and social psychological/sociological literatures in this section.
2 As Ferem notes, "Walls can be symbols of containment, or safety, they can be used as borders, psychological barriers, or symbols of unity" (Ferem, 1964, p. 15).
3 An earlier version in a different context of some of this material in this section can be found in Marcus (2015).
4 For an inside look at two graffiti artists who painted on New York City subways, see Knoll (2022).
5 This being said, some have claimed that most graffiti have a wide range of themes that are not easily characterized or catalogued.
6 Graffiti is thus fundamentally about leaving one's mark in the world.

References

Akhtar, S. (2009). *Comprehensive Dictionary of Psychoanalysis*, London: Karnac.
Bettelheim, B. (1962). *Symbolic Wounds*. New York: Collier Books.
Collins, R, & Cooper, P.J., (2005). *The Power of the Story: Teaching through Storytelling* (2nd ed.), Long Grove, Il: Waveland.
Dundes, A. (1966). Here I sit: A study of American latrinalia. *Kroeber Anthropological Society Papers*, 34: 91–105.
Ferem, M. (1964). *Bathroom Graffiti*. New York: Mark Batty Publishers.
Gadpaille, W.J. (1974). Graffiti: Psychoanalytic implications. In L. Gross (ed.) *Sexual behavior: Current issues*. Flushing, NY: Spectrum, 73–83.
Harvey, H.B. (2012). *The Art of Storytelling: From Parents to Professionals* (Transcript Book). Chantilly: VA: The Great Courses.
Haslam, N. (2012). *Psychology in the Bathroom*. New York: Palgrave Macmillan.
Kinsey, A.C., Pomeroy, W.B., Martin, C.E., & Gebbard, P.H. (1953). *Sexual behavior in the human female*. Philadelphia: W.B. Saunders.
Knoll, C. (2022). For Two Graffiti Artists, New York Subway was a Deadly Magnet. *New York Times*, May 5.
Landy, E.E. & Steele, J.M. (1967). Graffiti as a function of building utilization. *Perceptual and Motor Skills*, 25, 711–712.
Lippman, D. (1999) *Improving Your Storytelling: Beyond the Basics for All Who Tell Stories in Work or Play*. Atlanta, GA: August House.
Lomas, H. (1973). Graffiti: Some Observations and Speculations. *Psychoanalytic Review*, 60, 71–89.
Lomas, H. (1976). Graffiti: Some Clinical Observations. *Psychoanalytic Review*, 63, 451–457.

Lomas, H. (1980). Graffiti: Some Additional clinical observations. *Psychoanalytic Review*, 67, 139–142.

Marcus, P. (2015). *Creating Heaven on Earth. The Psychology of Experiencing Immortality in Everyday Life.* London: Karnac.

Marcus, P. with Marcus, G. (2011). *Theatre as Life: Practical Wisdom Drawn From Great Acting Teachers, Actors and Actresses.* Milwaukee, WI: Marquette University Press.

The Oxford Pocket Dictionary of Current English (2000). Oxford, UK: Oxford University Press. Online edition.

Rorty, R. (1989). *Contingency, Irony and Solidarity.* New York: Cambridge University Press.

Rycroft, C. (1995). *A Critical Dictionary of Psychoanalysis.* London: Penguin.

Chapter 6

Toilet Humor

Three examples of rather unusual toilet humor were recently reported in a popular magazine:

A British man has transformed his ability to fart at will into a livelihood as the entertainer Mr. Methane. Paul Oldfield, 55, discovered his super power as a teen when he noticed during yoga he could suck in air on both ends of his body. He travels the world to show case his unusual talent and is known for performing popular songs by modifying the tone and pitch of his farts. One of his most popular parodies is Phil Collins' "In the Air Tonight." (*The Week*, 10/15/21, p. 12)[1]

North Korea initiated a campaign to coerce citizens to produce more human and animal excrement for fertilizing crops. Citizens who fail to meet their manure quota will be fined and not permitted into public food markets, the government mandated. (*The Week*, 1/21/22, p. 6)

A Japanese man opened a shop in Japan devoted to poop-themed products, from clothing to accessories. "I wanted to make poop something funny, not dirty," said the owner, who sold poop-themed T-shirts online prior to opening the Unco shop, named after the Japanese word for poop. His store has a guest book in which visitors draw poops and laugh. "It transcends language and culture," said the owner, "and creates universal laughter". (*The Week*, 1/9/22, p. 12)

Some people find the aforementioned anecdotes not particularly amusing, the first appears to be preposterous and unconvincing while the second is absurdly brutal. The third appears to be unbelievable.

DOI: 10.4324/9781003219705-6

The fact is that to most people most toilet humor is more "in your face," or crude and low-brow than these examples, and many people find such humor to be on the "lower end" of the humor continuum. For example, "Why don't they have any toilet paper in KFC? Because its finger licking good." However, as Freud noted, "Not everyone; is capable of the humorous attitude. It is a rare and precious gift, and many people are even without the capacity to enjoy humorous pleasure that is presented to them," including toilet humor (Freud, 1927, p. 166). Indeed, toilet humor is especially difficult to listen to or read because it is of questionable taste, fart jokes for example, are hard to take except in small doses, in certain contexts, for most people. And yet they can be very funny if one is open to them. For example, actress Sandra Bullock noted, "Poop humor is fun. If you do the toilet scenes well and commit to them, they can be really, really powerful"; Likewise, the actor and comedian Adrian Edmondson noted, "There is a lot of rubbish written about toilet humour – people saying it is childish and pretending it is beneath them – but there is no doubting the effectiveness of a really good willy joke" [penis] (https://www.brainy quote.com/topics/toilet-quotes_2, retrieved 1/26/22). The fact is that the odors, noises and sounds that emanate from behind the bathroom door have been a great motivator for jokes and even comedic songs. Also, worth remembering is that the average man farts about 15 times a day while the woman about 9 times on the way to generating over a quart of gas (Blank, 2010, p. 62). Chaucer, Swift and Shakespeare for example, have also referenced the scatological, giving it a literary importance and this mode of humor goes back to ancient times (e.g., Seneca and the pre-Socratics). So, if everyone is farting many times a day (and using the toilet once a day or more to excrete and urinate), why is it regarded in such negative personal and social terms by most people? And why is it a staple for many comedians and casual jokers?

In this chapter I want to focus on the subject of toilet, potty or scatological humor, and suggest that there is more to this form of humor than is usually realized by the average person. Such humor focuses on excrement and excretion, or more generally on human waste (e.g., vomit), in ways that tends to generate a sense of disgust in the listener or reader and yet amuse them at the same time. "That laugh is an act of rebellion" (Praeger, 2007, p. 191). Indeed, disgust (and shame and guilt it is often associated with) is such a big part of people's response to this kind of humor, we need to unpack it in a bit more detail, while still keeping in mind the listener's possible amusement. By disgust I mean it as psychoanalysts tend to think about it.

Summarizing the matter, Akhtar drawing from Otto Fenichel, defines disgust as

> a feeling of revulsion with three levels (1) a physiological response to be repelled by certain tastes and smells, (2) its use by the ego for defensive purposes, especially for warding off oral and anal drives; overly intense disgust reactions, however betray their character as "reaction formation" where the suppressed interest in faeces, for instance, occasionally breaks through to the surface, and (3) "neurotic attacks of disgust"... in which the ego is completely overwhelmed by the affect, which was intended for defensive purposes. Here disgust can become quite similar to guilt, especially when it is disgust with oneself.
>
> (Akhtar, 2009, p. 81)[2]

For our purposes the second point seems the most relevant for it emphasizes the defense and highlights the internal excitement in the expression of the wish. As Haslam points out, disgust and shame are intimately connected to people's preoccupations about their bodies, and specifically about the violation of societal norms having to do with the body's cleanliness and purity. That is, we tend to feel shame most profoundly when our bodies have dissatisfied us in a manner that compromises our purity or dignity, especially when our failure is public.[3] People tend to feel guilt, Haslam notes, when they harm others or violate their rights, links to specific acts and prompts us to make reparation, but it is shame that devalues the whole self and motivates us to conceal ourselves "or sink into the ground" (Haslam, 2012, p. 9). In truth shame and guilt often go together, and when disgust is the psychological context, it is hard to separate, let alone distinguish shame and guilt clinically speaking.

I will focus this chapter as follows: a word on the developmental aspects of toilet humor, that is, the role of such humor in children through adolescence and beyond. Next, I will provide a hypothesis on why such humor is funny to the adult, and why some adults can't appreciate such humor and might be better off if they could. Finally, I will suggest that toilet humor has something to teach us about the human condition, about our collective anxieties and fears, and the possibility of the "transcendentally human" (Garber, 2014). As the great historian and sociologist Louis Mumford noted, "Today, the degradation of the inner life is symbolized by the fact that the only place sacred from interruption is the private toilet" (https://www.brainyquote.com/topics/toilet-quotes_2, retrieved 1/26/22). In other words, the toilet is like a fallout shelter, a person's last refuge where he reminds himself that he is still a human being (Ferem, 1964).

Before doing so, I want to succinctly state the overarching focus of this chapter, best captured by Deirdre Kay on the internet, who has collected many of the best examples of toilet humor out there in the public domain:

> Something smells, and it smells bad. Must be the odor of these funny poop jokes and puns? No matter your age, a good poop and diarrhea joke will always bring the kid out in you. After all, it's the great equalizer, isn't it? We all poop! For decades, poop jokes have reigned supreme as the funniest jokes to crack (pun intended). We're pretty sure our parents and their parents' parents told a poop (or a fart) joke or two. The point is, poop jokes are classic, and so we've gathered all the funnies you'll need to keep this tradition going.
>
> Gone are the days you had to stifle your laugh in class or in front of your mother because someone passed gas. This is your time to laugh hard and valiantly because poop jokes were and will always be hilarious. We know that pooping is a little gross to talk about or bring up at the dinner table, but giggling about the things that pop out of our bodies has always had its own special brand of comedy. We've known this since we were children and they're just as funny today as they were then.

Moreover, says Kay, her collecting various toilet humor examples, is meant to help the adult reconnect to that child inside so that he may one day pass it on to his own inappropriate children! (https://www.sca rymommy.com/poop-jokes/, retrieved 1/22/22).

Toilet Humor in Children

How children develop a sense of humor is a huge topic in the psychological literature, but a word about it seems necessary to understand the likely origins of toilet humor. Church (2022, np), provides a neat summary of development from birth through age 6. What is most important for us, is when the child becomes interested in toilet humor.

In stage 0 to 2, says Church, a baby's reactions to playful physical interchanges are his first steps toward what we call humor. For example, bouncing and tickling, body contact that generates laughs, wiggles, and smiles. Also, parent noises that are unexpected can amuse the infant. Interesting sounds fascinate infants. Memory and imitation help 1-year-olds sort out that it is funny to do something unanticipated like playing peek-a-boo. A toddler's often creative use of symbols and language contributes to them playing with reality. Incongruities are particularly funny (there is an Incongruity theory of humor in the literature), such as a 2-year old joking that Daddy eats chairs, or Daddy eats poop. In stage 3 to 4, the 3-year-old likes sharing their sense of humor with important adults like parents and teachers. Pre-schoolers enjoy creating silly and ridiculous stories. However, it is 4-year-olds who "are fascinated by bathroom humor and are not completely sensitive to the effect their humor has on others" (ibid), including using it to attack, "you're a poop head." It is through such humor that they learn for instance, the limitations of their bodies, and to delineate the social construction of normality, that is, they learn what is permissible and not permissible (Blank, 2010).

As Marder (2020), citing psychologist Lawrence Cohen notes, bodily functions are especially strong in young children at this stage which is connected to the words that are used to describe them. There is a strong sensory experience of using the bathroom, amalgamated with "the hush-hush" privacy and secrecy that children notice as adults respond to their words. Thus, children acquire a degree of power that they did not have, when they see their parents and caregivers be awkward, nervously laugh or in other ways respond to the child's provocative words. Toilet humor in young children is thus appealing because the child feels empowered. These considerations in part, account for the fact that children can run around the house saying the word "poop" or its variations out loud which provokes in them hysterical laughter.

Young children, writes Marder, also use toilet humor to work through their many anxieties associated with the bathroom experience like having an accident or so-called castration anxiety ("there is a crocodile in the toilet" my 3-year-old son told me). In other words, since the toilet is a place of many accidents generating anxiety in the child who is being toilet trained (about 2 to 4), making toilet jokes helps them master their anxiety and reduces their tensions, Marder says (citing Laura Markham and Dorris Bergen, both researchers into children's humor). Such behavior tends to be socially acceptable to the young child, though not to the often, frustrated adult. One only has to think of adult comedians who often joke about their worst experiences as children, in a sense they are mastering their traumas by joking about them. Age 4 is also a time when the child develops a good sense of humor which conveys a wide range of emotions, including highly negative ones that could almost never be expressed directly. Thus, the "good enough" parent probes the "deeper" meaning of what the child says in terms of the child's unconscious needs and wishes.

In stage 5 to 6, says Church, 5- and 6-year-olds' vocabularies have evolved to the point where they can play with substituting words in a sentence to recognize the humor in it. Kindergartners also develop motor skills that allow them to play with being uncoordinated as a way of sharing humor. Five- and 6-year-olds exploit humor as a way of creating friendships and becoming part of the larger group. Such social bonding jokes becomes progressively elaborated as the child gets older and moves into adolescence and young adulthood. For example, in adolescence toilet humor includes jokes about sexuality, gender, politics, nationality and the like.

Thus, it would seem that toilet humor begins in the anal phase but consolidates around the Oedipal stage about age 4 to 5, the preschool years. This is when the child is being, or has been toilet trained but is still sensitive to the happenings in the bathroom, for him, and his caregivers. What we want to understand is how such humor is transposed to adulthood. How such early humor grounded in two early prohibitions, anal and Oedipal, continues to have an impact on adult humor.

Toilet Humor in Adults

Adult humor thus requires the ability to consciously or unconsciously call to mind something of the experience of the preschool years in order to be funny, or at least amusing. To understand why toilet humor is funny, we need to know something about the function of humor in adult life, from a psychoanalytic point of view.

Briefly, for Freud (1905), the main thrust of jokes included the following: (1) aesthetic pleasure that gives way to a transient weakening of repression and the discharge of sublimated energy; (2) there is a greater significance to form than content in terms of how the story is narrated; (3) similar to dreams (but differently too) there is a use of condensation, displacement, reversal and the fusion of instincts; (4) by-passing the censorship due to the disguise of the instinctual aims (Akhtar, 2009, p. 155). Thus, the joke is funny. Freud believed that humor was a "triumph of narcissism," "the victorious assertion of the ego's invulnerability" in the face of suffering (Freud, 1927, p. 162).[4]

There are a number of theories of humor. Relief theory alleges that laughter is a homeostatic mechanism by which psychological stress and tension is diminished. The incongruity theory alleges that humor emerges at the point of realization of incongruity between a concept operative in a specific situation and the real objects conceived in some relation or linkage to the concept. Superiority theory alleges that a person laughs at the bad luck and failings of others because these failures express the person's superiority in the context of the bad luck and failings of others. Freud believed that the mechanism at work was the energic tension is accumulated as a person represses his hostility, anxiety or sexual desire that is socially inappropriate to express. A clever or witty remark stimulates a release of that energy through laughter, specifically when the clever or witty comment relates to the person or situation that stimulated the hostility, anxiety or desire (Spiegel, 2013, p. 19). That is, the joke or witty comment is relieving the expression of the repressed wish. Freud's view is thus an example of Relief theory.

An example of these aforementioned dynamics at least in part comes from Winston Churchill who had a famous one-line toilet joke: "When he was disturbed from his 'thinking time in the throne' by a call from Lord Privy Seal, Churchill easily responded with '*Tell him I can only deal with one shit at a time*'"(Khodaiji, 2019, n.p.). In this somewhat atypical toilet joke we see the hostile wish directed at Lord Seal while at the same time the play on words acts as the defense, in other words, it softens the blow of the hostile comment. Incongruity is also at work in this example, the great Churchill on the toilet conducting official business.

Farting

Moving from Freud's general theory of humor we come to what is a universal phenomenon, namely, farting. For most people it generates amusement, for others it can produce embarrassment, and for the unfortunate few it can be nothing short of a horrible burden (Haslam, 2012, p. 52). Farting has been the source of many jokes by professional comedians. As George Carlin noted about his famous comedy show: "Where would a comedy show be without a few fart jokes." Indeed, there are some good reasons why something we all do every day is funny in certain contexts (https://www.speeli.com, Humor, retrieved 4/8/22).

First, fart jokes are unanticipated, that is, unexpected. Think of the fart that accidentally occurs in a church for all to hear, and why it is funny. It is incongruous with the situation (Incongruity theory), it releases tension (Relief theory), and it gives the audience a sense of superiority compared to the poor soul who has embarrassed himself (Superiority theory). Sometimes the farter deliberately farts in the church and his expression of hostility gives him a perverse sense of superiority to the other worshippers and clergy (ibid.).

Second, farters use humor to conceal and disguise their embarrassment. That is, they use humor to reduce the intensity of this undesirable emotion. When a person is embarrassed because he has unexpectedly farted, he can almost immediately use humor to improve his mood and in his mind, ease the condemnation of others who smell the fart (ibid.)

Third, farting breaks the rules of normal and acceptable conduct. It violates taboos and is fundamentally subversive. This is why children, especially teenagers, like to do it. It is rule-breaking activity that is funny (ibid.).

Fourth, a fart is usually funnier if people feel they are trapped. For example, if it happened inside an automobile, lift or enclosed waiting room then the one who did it might find it very funny and because humor is transmittable others might respond with laughter. Farts tend to be funnier when they are done among friends compared to complete strangers (ibid.).

Fifth, while both boys and girls can find farts funny still the near universal stereotype set for girls, that they should be well-mannered and reticent, can inhibit girls from laughing at farts as much as boys do. This may account for why researchers claim that in general, women fart less than men. (ibid.).

Sixth, farts can occasionally be enigmatic because it can be difficult to discern who dealt it, especially given the fact that sometimes people keep denying that they did them. "Whoever dealt it, smelt it" the popular saying goes. People have been conditioned to find farts funny, a kind of learned behavior from for example, parents and the social media. The fact that farts are linked in people's minds with fun in many contexts make them funnier to many people. And it is noteworthy and there are hundreds of fart jokes circulating in our society. As I said, farting and fart jokes appear to be a subject in every culture and historical epoch (ibid.).

Seventh, in some contexts, farts help the person achieve the unconscious wish to punish some of his friends or retaliate against them. This usually occurs with children, especially teenagers. The fact that the fart helps the child (or adult) meet a desired goal tends to make it more satisfying and fun (ibid.).

Eighth, farts can release stress and tension because they can be considered an immature behavior, child's play (Relief theory). When an adult person does something immature without hurting anybody, he relieves some of the tension of being so serious all the time (ibid.).

Ninth, for some reason, the fact that farts come from the rear end makes them funnier than burping which comes from the mouth. Farts carry the weight of being especially disgusting and rule and taboo-breaking compared to say burping. This is probably because the taboo on anal phase material is stronger than on the oral phase material like burping which is much more socially acceptable (ibid.).

Tenth, it should always be remembered that fart jokes are context-dependent and setting specific. That is, a fart joke can be very funny in certain situations such as in church or when a comedian makes a fart joke, versus a fart during a job interview or during a colonoscopy (ibid.).

All of the aforementioned characteristics which detail why and how fart humor is funny draw from different theories. However, it is Spiegel's (2013) theory which seems most inclusive and plausible, generally speaking. For example, he notes that not only does this theory support the insights of the three major theories of humor, but it accounts for something that none of the theories can explain, namely, laughter that results from tickling, particularly of infants and young toddlers. That is, says Spiegel, children and toddlers are cognitively too immature to perceive incongruities or to have a genuine sense of self, much less the capacity to a feeling of comparative superiority. They are also too immature to have the social awareness required to produce the nervous energy requisite for laughter on this account (ibid., p. 20).

Spiegel provides an interesting explanation why flatulence is funny. Drawing from the work of religious philosopher John Morreall who discerns a common thread among the three theories of humor, Spiegel claims that the

> common core to each of the major views, [is] namely the notion that laughter always results from a "pleasant psychological shift" of some kind. Incongruity theorists focus on the cognitive forms that this shift often takes, while superiority and relief theorists emphasize affective dimensions. But for there to be true humor, and ultimately laughter as a physical response, this psychological shift must be *pleasant*.
>
> (Spiegel, 2013, p. 20)

Thus, Spiegel believes that farting is funny because it satisfies the psychological conditions for humor, that is, it generates laughter because it produces the pleasant psychological shift. The pleasant psychological shift in the aforementioned infant tickling example is physical or purely perceptual in nature. Says Spiegel, "whether tickling or making faces at an infant or young toddler, the child surely experiences a 'pleasant psychological shift', so the consequent laughter is easily accounted for" (i.e., Morreall's fundamental concept has strong explanatory power). (ibid.). Flatulence is also funny because it produces a sudden upsurge of felt superiority. As a social taboo, passing gas signifies a lack of self-control and, thus, diminished dignity. It is also funny because it provides multiple incongruities and prompts laughter because being socially taboo in most contexts, it gives a release of nervous energy in the form of laughter among those who witness it. Summarizing his perspective, Spiegel concludes that farting "is a phenomenon that prompts a sudden sense of superiority, is incongruous with many aspects of human social life, and creates a constant exertion of mental energy from which we all need relief from time to time" (ibid., p. 24).[5]

In passing, it should be mentioned that some people have what is called "joke blindness," what often appears to be a defect in the brain, characterized by truncated empathy that prevents them from getting the joke. Such people are humorless because they are so defended from amusing affects which they experience as threatening. These people miss out on a whole domain of enjoyment of toilet and other forms of humor.

Bowel Movement, Constipation, Diarrhea and Peeing Jokes

There are other types of toilet humor where the focus is not on farting, but on other expressions of excretory distress. Below are a few examples with brief commentary why these jokes and witticisms are possibly funny. I have not dealt with so-called "dirty jokes," even though Freud alleged that infantile play with excrement expresses itself in its adult form in the telling of "dirty jokes" (Freud, 1905, pp. 97–98).

A blonde goes to the doctor because she couldn't make a bowel movement. The doctor prescribes a suppository and sends her on her way. She returns a week later complaining the laxative did not work.
Doctor: Have you been taking them regularly?
Blonde: What do you think I've been doing, shoving them up my ass?
(https://upjoke.com/bowel-movement-jokes, retrieved 2/1/22)

The punchline is funny because it highlights the "shock and horror" of having to put suppositories up one's rear end. The graphic language cuts through the defenses of the listener against their discomfort with suppositories. What also makes this joke funny is that it plays with the listener's expectations, taking the suppositories regularly, and then the punch line corrects the miscommunication and/or defense, but with a hostile edge.

> I went to the doctor because I hadn't had a bowel movement in nearly 2 weeks. The doctor says to me:
> "Well, it sounds like you're really bunged up."
> I replied "No shit!"
>
> (ibid)

Here the listener smiles in part, because the patient is making fun of the banal words of the doctor, again with a hostile edge. However, more profoundly, this joke's answer to the problem of constipation provides an accurate description of the condition ("no shit") and with a hostile response to the banality of the doctor's response.

> Three old men were sitting around and talking. The 80 year-old said, "The best thing that could happen to me would just to be able to have a good pee. I stand there for twenty minutes, and it dribbles and hurts. I have to go over and over again." The 85 year-old said, "The best thing that could happen to me is if I could have one good bowel movement. I take every kind of laxative I can get my hands on and it's still a problem." Then the 90 year-old said, "That's not my problem. Every morning at 6:00 am sharp, I have a good long pee. At 6:30 am sharp I have a great bowel movement. The best thing that could happen to me would be if I could wake up before 7:00 am.
>
> (ibid.)

While the joke firsts details the typical mishaps of old age around peeing and taking a bowel movement, generating our empathy for the old folks, the punch line in effect says, it is even worse than you imagined this getting old business. That is, we are all going to get decrepit, sick and die and the punchline bypasses the defense against the fear of getting old, hence it is amusing.

> Did you hear about the constipated mathematician? He worked it out with a pencil.
> (https://worstjokesever.com/constipation, retrieved 1/2/22).

This joke is amusing because it is so disgusting, though familiar to anyone who has been constipated where they are forced to use their fingers to release the feces that is distressing them. That is, the joke violates the defense against the "secret" that sometimes such anal or rectal digging is necessary.

What did the left butt cheek say to the right butt cheek?
"Together we can stop this shit!"

(ibid.)

This diarrhea joke simply plays with one's fantasy wish that the diarrhea would stop. It is the imagined relief that is amusing as if the redemption is in the person's control.

Have you heard about the movie Constipation?
No, Because It never came out...

(ibid.)

This joke is a play on words, taking the literality of a movie coming out and juxtaposing it with the wish of the constipated person to have a bowel movement.

How do you help a constipated person?
You scare the shit out of them.

(ibid.)

This joke is funny because it plays with the hostile wish to coerce a constipated person into a normal bowel movement. That is, the hostile though ultimately benign wish to "scare the shit" out of someone is made acceptable, at least for a moment, and this makes us laugh.

Conclusion

What makes toilet humor funny, at least in part, is its subversive nature. That is, it seeks out the "rebellious" in human behavior (Freud, 1927, p. 163). Praeger further notes, that scatological humor, "invokes the disgust surrounding the body's waste products for laughs. That laugh is an act of rebellion" (Praeger, 2007, pp. 192–193). Citing the French sociologist Pierre Bourdieu, compared to high culture, popular culture was described as "a refusal of the refusal which is the starting point of high aesthetic" (ibid., p. 192). Praeger extends Bourdieu's analysis and makes the following important point:

Laughing at scatological humor means rejecting the mandate to reject poop. In potty training, you learned that the rules of society sometimes require the rejection of the desires of the body. To reject the rejection, you're rebelling against the potty-training-instilled foundations of the rules of society.

(ibid.)

For example, while farting in the bathroom is permissible it is not acceptable in a house of worship. If you consent to something knowing it's unacceptable, you are in effect refusing the refusal that the rules and prohibitions of society command. "Scatological humor presents poop in situations in which you know you're supposed to refuse it. Laughing at a fart in church is a refusal of that refusal. It's a rebellion against the voice of civilization—against society" (ibid.). As Praeger notes, adolescents love scatological humor less because they are immature and more because they identify with the subversive nature of toilet humor. While old folks and those in authority regard toilet humor as threatening to their authoritative role in society (ibid.). Two simple examples told to me by an internet surfing teenager who had oppositional and defiant tendencies:

1) What is the true definition of bravery?
Chancing a fart when you know you have diarrhea.
2) Why didn't the soldier flush the toilet?
It wasn't his duty.
(https://www.scarymommy.com/poop-jokes/, retrieved 2/2/22)

Thus, there's a tension between liking and disliking toilet jokes as one grows older. As I noted, children like toilet jokes as a way of coping with the magnitude and power of a new experience. One doesn't hear "people of class" making these kinds of jokes, which is why when one hears them, they are awkward and embarrassing to many people. It would be interesting for researchers to further explore whether there is a certain personality type that tells these jokes, who likes them and who doesn't. Making fun of something so personal and private is one of the reasons why people like these jokes as well as dislike them. The jokes bring us into a realm of the forbidden which is why they can be appealing.

Finally, given that toilet humor is a sub-species of humor in general, it shares some of the characteristics of humor that are in play when humor is used in psychotherapy (Martin, 2007). The following descriptions although used to highlight the use of humor in psychotherapy are a very clear elaboration of some of the mechanisms that are deployed in toilet humor.

Indeed, Freud advocated the judicious use of lighthearted and skillful humor during sessions, and he was known to have a good sense of humor, especially his affection for "Jewish" jokes. As Lemma (2000, p. 154) notes humor, and to some extent this includes toilet humor, promotes introspection and an observing ego. This includes the internalization of a model of intrapsychic communication which improves mood and reduces anxiety; it permits interpretation by bypassing resistance, that is, humor expresses the wish without interfering defensiveness; humor especially toilet humor, tends to focus on themes which evoke anxiety, and therefore it helps the person moderate his anxiety and strengthens the ego; it tends to lift repression and comforts, while acknowledging the hold on the patient of internal conflict and outer distress; humor, says Lemma, modulates the superego by promoting its benign elements. More particularly, if humor is used in therapy it strengthens the therapeutic alliance in that laughing together solidifies a relationship. It also puts into sharp focus the analyst's ability to tolerate and master certain emotions and roles brought about by the patient's projective processes. This includes the analyst's willingness and ability to affectionately recognize the patient's hostility, as well as affirm his wish to establish mutuality of a sort; lastly, says Lemma, humor "undermines fixed or habitual views and attitudes by introducing alternative or unexpected options" (ibid.). Toilet humor, like all humor is therefore, an act of emotional "problem solving" and tends to expand and deepen consciousness, this being one of the important goals of psychoanalysis.

Notes

1 There have been other similar entertainers before Oldfield cited in the literature.
2 There has been an upsurge of disgust interest in social psychology, but for our purposes we mean it from a psychoanalytic point of view.
3 One of the best definitions of shame comes from Alissa Bennett, who wrote that "the primary social function of shame—often a tool of oppression and always one that aims to police those who bear witness—is to neutralize transgression via humiliation, to force consensus by threat of moral exile" (Bennett, 2022).
4 See my study of tragic comic humor as it relates to the art of living a flourishing life (Marcus, 2013).
5 Farting can get you into big trouble too. For example, star Brazilian defender Marcelo was dropped from French soccer club Lyon for repeatedly farting and laughing in the dressing room after a loss (*The Week*, 5/20/2022).

References

Akhtar, S. (2009). *Comprehensive Dictionary of Psychoanalysis*. London: Karnac.

Bennett, A. (2022). No Pain, No Gain. Who wins in our culture of public excoriation? *New York Times Book Review*, p. 21. May 8.

Blank, J.J. (2010). Cheeky Behavior: The meaning and function of "Fartlore" in childhood and adolescence. *Children's Folklore and Review*, 32, 61–85.

Church, E.B. (2022.). Ages & Stages: Don't forget to laugh! The importance of humor. https://www.scholastic.com/teachers/articles/teaching-content/a ges-stages-dont-forget-laugh-importance-humor/ (retrieved 1/27/22).

Ferem, M. (1964). *Bathroom Graffti*. New York: Mark Battery Publisher.

Freud, S. (1927). Humour. *The Standard Edition of the Complete Psychological Works of Sigmund Freud*, Trans J. Strachey with A. Freud assisted by A. Stratchey and A. Tyson, 24 volumes (1953–1974). London: Hogarth Press and the Institute of Psycho-Analysis, vol. 21, 161–172. (Henceforth *S.E.*).

Freud, S. (1905). Jokes and their relation to the unconscious. *S.E.* 8, 9–236.

Garber, M. (2014). The World is Flatulence: The Enduring Appeal Of The Tasteless. *The Atlantic*. https://www.theatlantic.com, retrieved 1/26/22.

Haslam, N. (2012). *Psychology in the Bathroom*. New York: Palgrave Macmillan.

Khodaiji, D.M. (2019). Remembering Winston Churchill and his Wit! https://parsi-times.com/2019/01/remembering-winston-and-his-wit/ (retrieved 1/31/22).

Lemma, A. (2000). *Humour on the Couch. Exploring Humour in Psychotherapy and Everyday Life*. London: Whurr Publishers.

Marcus, P. (2013). *How to laugh your way through life*. London: Karnac.

Marder, J (2020). Why are kids so obsessed with poop jokes. Toilet humor can be a powerful too for children, but there are ways to limit the potty talk. *New York Times*, May 4. https://www.nytimes.com/2020/04/15/parenting/kids-potty-humor.html (retrieved 1/27/22).

Martin, R.A. (2007). *The Psychology of Humor: An Integrative Approach*. Amsterdam: Elsevier.

Praeger, D. (2007). *Poop Culture. How America is Shaped By Its Grossest National Product*. Los Angeles, CA: Feral House.

Spiegel, J.S. (2013). Why flatulence is funny. *Think*, 12, 35, 15–24.

The Week (2021). It must be true...I read it in the tabloids. October 15, 12.

The Week (2022). Good week for:. January 22, 6.

The Week (2022). Bad week for:. May 20, 6.

The Week (2022). It must be true...I read it in the tabloids. September 9, 12.

Chapter 7

The Personal Meaning of Urinating and Defecating

It seems fitting that in the last chapter of this book, we deal with the personal meaning of urinating and defecating in situations that are both distressing, such as the consequences of having an enlarged prostate or being subjected to "excremental assault" in the Nazi concentration camps, and positively perplexing, as when a person dreams about urine or excrement. As I discussed adult female urinary incontinence in Chapter Three, this chapter will focus on problems specific to men.

Enlarged prostate

As urologist Stephen Summers points out (2022, n.p.), frequently in one's 40s or 50s a man may notice that he is awakened more often at night to go to the toilet. This occurrence is often due to prostate enlargement, a problem that does not easily go away and may morph into prostate cancer. In general, an enlarged prostate gets worse as one gets older. It is estimated that about 50 percent of men have what is called Benign prostatic hyperplasia (BPH), a condition in which the prostate gland grows inward and presses on the urethra, impeding the urinary system (ibid.). Investigators do not know why prostate enlargement occurs, it tends to be genetic but other contributing elements include obesity, high blood sugar, and high intake of caffeine and alcohol, both of which irritate the bladder (ibid.). The typical symptoms of BPH are says Summers, a slow stream of urine, starting and stopping while urinating, a difficulty emptying one's bladder completely, bladder irritation and discomfort, feeling an urgency to urinate, awakening many times at night to urinate and/or urinary incontinence (ibid.) While there are some medicinal and surgical treatments available for these symptoms (though some lead to erectile dysfunction and other problems) what I want to focus on is the

DOI: 10.4324/9781003219705-7

personal psychological meaning of these symptoms in terms of how a man relates to his penis during the toileting experience.

However, before commenting on the meaning of the above symptoms to the typical man, it is necessary to explain two psychoanalytic notions: Freud's (1925) idea of phallic narcissism or phallic pride as Wilhelm Reich called it, "refers to the euphoria and self-infatuation that boys display in 'discovering' their penises" (Akhtar, 2009, p. 208). However, soon their interest in the penis is displaced to lengthened objects, such as toys in the form of racing cars, airplanes, knives guns, and activities and fantasies that include the penis (ibid.). As Akhtar further notes, the near manic-like excitement the child feels also commemorates the avenue of flight from symbiotic engulfment by the mother (or main caregiver) since the penis affirms being dissimilar to the mother and acts as a defensive regime against intense castration anxiety. Over time, says Akhtar, the autoerotic phallic narcissism slowly evolves into more object-relatedness as the child progresses into the oedipal phase. However, relics of phallic narcissism might remain throughout life, giving the adult character a "cocky" and exhibitionistic tendency (ibid). It is important to recognize that in phallic narcissism, it is aggression that dominates over eroticism, and its superordinate goal is for self-aggrandizement rather than discharge (Moore & Fine, 1990).

Urethral eroticism, what Freud (1905) earlier called urinary eroticism, is a notion that relates to the pleasure derived from urination. Both excretory and retentive pleasures are in play in relation to urination. Largely autoerotic, urethral eroticism soon morphs to include objects and gets linked with fantasies about urinating "at objects, being urinated on by objects, or with fantasies" in which the linkage with urination is more hidden (Akhtar, 2009, p. 303, he is quoting Otto Fenichel). Urethral eroticism, says Akhtar, can have active and passive modes of expression. The active mode of expression comprises "pleasures of forcefully urinating to damage something, to make it wet, to put a fire out, to compete with others about the strength and duration of the urinary stream" (as is so common with children and teenagers) (ibid.). The passive mode of expression comprises the pleasures of gently surrendering urinary control and relinquishing any sense of agency for the act. "The active form of urethral eroticism, especially in boys, frequently becomes condensed with phallic penetrative fantasies, and the passive form with anal receptive aims or fantasies of being a woman" (ibid.). In girls, the notion of letting the urine flow passively is occasionally displaced upwards and causes frequent tearfulness. In both sexes, loss of bladder control is closely connected with shame, which, in some instances, is defended against by ambition, through clearly ambition emanates from diverse childhood sources (ibid.).

As I said, following Summers, the typical symptoms of BPH are, (1) a slow stream of urine, (2) starting and stopping while urinating, (3) a difficulty emptying one's bladder completely, (4) bladder irritation and discomfort, (5) feeling an urgency to urinate, and (6) awakening many times at night to urinate and/or urinary incontinence. These symptoms may have different meanings for different individuals however, in describing some of the feelings evoked by these symptoms in some of my patients I hope to convey how undermining the symptoms can be to a person's sense of self-continuity, self-esteem and self-cohesion.

1   A slow stream of urine can connote a lack of power and potency compared to when one was young. It calls to mind the games that children and young teenagers sometimes play where they compete to see who can urinate the furthest.

2   Starting and stopping while urinating can signify a lack and loss of control over something that was always taken for granted, the very quality of a person that provides him with a sense of self-efficacy and self-respect.

3   A difficulty emptying one's bladder completely also can signify a lack of control and inadequacy. This inability to empty one's bladder and the powerlessness inherent in that may stir up feelings of castration—the penis just doesn't work.

4   Bladder irritation and discomfort often causes anger and irritability not only because of the pain, but also because of anger at one's penis and associated bad "plumbing," a feeling that one is powerless to change.

5   Feeling an urgency to urinate, with the danger of actually wetting oneself, can lead to a profound sense of loss of control along with a sense of being both ashamed and guilty at one's state.

6   Awakening many times at night to urinate and/or urinary incontinence can evoke the loss of control over one's body and a lack of potency or virility at being at the mercy of one's bladder.

In terms of phallic narcissism these symptoms represent an assault on any sense of phallic pride a man may have. As one older patient of mine told me, "it just hangs there, and I have to piss all the time which is very uncomfortable." Likewise, these symptoms undermine the man's healthy sense of urethral eroticism, because the symptoms are all a downward modification of prior functioning giving the man the sense that he was not what he was when he was younger and more virile.

A brief word on prostate cancer seems pertinent. It has been estimated that every year about half a million men are diagnosed with prostate cancer in the US and Europe (Scholz & Blum, 2021). Put differently, according to the American Cancer Society, in 2017, it was estimated that there were about 161,360 new cases of prostate cancer in the U.S. and 26,730 related deaths (Vartolomei et al, 2018). Most importantly, this disease impacts one's quality of life and this can include the daily experience of urinating. For example, a large amount of men reports urinary problems as a side effect of their treatment. This is due to the fact that prostate cancer treatment (surgery, radiation and drugs) can damage the nerves and muscles that control when you urinate causing all types of urinating problems. Some of the symptoms of prostate cancer are an exacerbated version of those men who have an enlarged prostate have, though blood in the urine from surgery, radiation or drugs is not uncommon, causing anxiety and fear in the man. To suggest that blood in the urine can stir up castration anxiety is obvious just as erectile dysfunction can, the latter being a somewhat common consequence of surgery, radiation and drugs.

It should be mentioned that there are about 75,000 radical prostatectomies performed every year in the US, though more than 40,000 are unnecessary (Scholz & Blum, 2021), which suggests that watchful waiting or active surveillance is often a better approach to non-aggressive prostate cancer. Active surveillance means "active observation and regular monitoring of a patient without actual treatment" (ibid., p. 167). Many men die of other causes before prostate cancer metastasizes and kills them.

As to the management of prostate cancer in terms of urination problems (Martins, 2022) non-invasive recommendations are somewhat similar to women who have urinary incontinence (see Chapter Three). They too, require a refashioning of everyday habits, often causing anxiety and the like. For example, patients may find it helpful scheduling their urination every three and a half hours or so while awake even if they don't feel the need to go to the toilet. Patients who are unable to completely empty their bladder, says Martins, may attempt a procedure called double voiding, by relaxing for a short time and urinating again. Discomfort may be diminished by making an easy-to-access and quicker path to the bathroom, in addition to wearing clothes easier to take off such as elastic waistbands or Velcro fasteners, and by keeping a urinal close by. Other recommendations that may enhance the patient's health include not smoking, and having a healthy diet and weight, physical exercise and so on (ibid.). What should appear obvious to the reader, is whether it is due to the disease or treatment (surgery, radiation, drugs), the negative impact of having prostate cancer on a man's narrative of self-identity can be profound, and this includes being reminded of his troubling circumstances while urinating. Learning to live with the disease in terms of watchful waiting or active surveillance, or submitting to surgery, radiation and/or drugs, puts a huge burden on a man's ability to maintain his self-efficacy, self-esteem and self-respect. In this context, going to the toilet to urinate can be nothing short of an ordeal of suffering.

Excremental Assault in the Nazi Death Camps

It was Terrence Des Pres who used the evocative term "excremental assault" in his masterpiece *The Survivor. An Anatomy of Life in the Death Camps* (1976). The term has been described as follows:

> In Nazi camps especially, dirt and excrement were permanent conditions of existence. In the barracks at night, for example, "buckets of excrement stood in a little passage by the exit. There were not enough. By dawn the whole floor was awash with urine and feces. We carried the filth about the hut on our feet, the stench made people faint".
>
> (ibid, p. 53, Des Pres is quoting a survivor)

Indeed, Des Pres catalogues in painful detail the fact "that prisoners were *systematically* subjected to filth. They were the deliberate target of excremental assault" (ibid., p. 57). Moreover, the prisoner's subjection to filth caused more despair than hunger or fear of dying (ibid, p. 66).

Des Pres makes the important point that the Nazis could have killed a prisoner whenever he wanted and yet, the death of the prisoner was the penultimate goal. Rather before they were murdered they needed to be crushed as self-respecting human beings. "Excremental assault, the physical inducement of disgust and self-loathing was a principle weapon" of the prisoner's dehumanization (ibid., p. 60). "Spiritual destruction became an end in itself, quite apart from the requirements of mass murder" (ibid.). By degrading the prisoner, the SS made the prisoner into a humiliated object: "How much self-esteem can one maintain, how readily can one respond with respect to the needs of another [fellow inmates], if both stink, if both are caked with mud and feces" (and have diarrhea, no nearby toilet and no toilet paper) (ibid). Des Pres quotes one survivor who puts the point just right:

> They condemned us to die in our own filth, to drown in mud, in our own excrement. They wished to abase us, to destroy our human dignity, to efface every vestige of humanity, to return to the level of wild animals, to fill us with horror and contempt toward ourselves and our fellows.
>
> (ibid, p. 63)

I could go on and give many more examples of excremental assault from Des Pres's book but the point I want to emphasize is this: Excrement, something we all have inside us, can be used as the ultimate degrader of the human being. In fact, Des Pres describes one of the strangest instances when defilement caused a personal breakdown that bordered on madness. He describes the scenario when a collection of prisoners was forced to drink out of the prison toilet bowls. Quoting a survivor, Des Pres writes

> The men could not bring themselves to obey this devilish order; they only pretended to drink. But the block fuehrers had reckoned with that; they forced the men's heads deep into the bowls until their faces were covered with excrement. At this the victims went out of their minds—that was why their screams had sounded so demented.
>
> (ibid., p. 66)

Des Pres further asks the question why is contact with excrement utterly intolerable? That is, if the actual experience of being in contact with excrement in terms of discomfort is relatively minor, why was the reaction to the drinking out of toilet bowls so violent?

Des Pres considers it implausible to attribute the pain of these prisoners to a violation of a cultural taboo as some analyst's believed. Rather, he claims, and I agree with him, that the answer to these questions has something to do with what Paul Ricoeur called "dread of the impure" (1967, p. 41, quoted from Des Pres). Des Pres says that when civilization breaks down as it did in the camps, the prisoner was denuded of his expanded spiritual identity and only concrete forms of existence were in play, "actual life and actual death, actual pain and actual defilement," (ibid., p. 68) and these now composed the vehicle of moral and spiritual being. With the prisoner reduced to the corporeal experience of his body, the literal defilement and evil becomes that which cause the disintegration of the sense of self, who they were or had been in a previous life before their incarceration. That is, excremental assault was a threat that went beyond suffering and death because it tried to diminish existence to cause a loss of the person's moral/spiritual core of their way of being-in-the-world. The aforementioned prisoners were thus, not responding to what excrement symbolizes, rather their ordeal of suffering was the concrete moment from which the symbolism of evil emanated (ibid., p. 68).

Defecation and Urination Dreams

Defecation and urination dreams are very common among analysands, and people in general, again emphasizing the importance of excrement and urine in human psychological experience. While Freud regarded dreams as the "royal road" to understanding the unconscious, the probable meaning of a dream can only be found via the analysand's associations to parts of the dream. Even then, there is always more that can be made of a dream than what the analyst and the analysand "agree" is the likely meaning of the dream. Freud (1900) mentioned that there are "dreams of convenience" such as tension-reducing dreaming about going to the toilet when one has a full bowel. This being said, defecation and urination dreams have many meanings, and they tend to exemplify the work of symbolism in a relatively clear manner. Freud, in his Rat Man case mentions a dream the patient had. "He dreamt that he saw my daughter in front of him; she had two patches of dung instead of eyes." Freud commented, "No one who understands the language of dreams will find much difficulty in translating this one: it declared that he was marrying my daughter not for her 'beaux yeux' [beautiful eyes] but for her money" (Freud, 1909, p. 200). What follows are three clinical vignettes of analysands who had a defecation and urination dreams.

Vignette One

Avi, in his late 60s, was the son of two Jewish Holocaust survivors. He was happily married and had three children all who sounded rather accomplished in their work and happy in their family lives. Avi was a successful electrical engineer and had his own consulting firm. He came to me because he was depressed and anxious about getting old, sick and dying, and learning to live more effectively with a chronic painful disability (inoperable back pain). I had been seeing Avi twice a week for about two years, he was a cooperative and articulate patient who was prone to feeling guilty and ashamed for neurotic reasons, connected we thought to his two survivor parents both who had died in the last few years. In the transference I was usually perceived as a benign father figure, though Avi had a bad temper and if I said something that he felt was "dumb" or unhelpful, he could get very angry and retaliatory at my imperfections. Below was Avi's defecation dream.

> I dreamt that I was wandering lost in a dark forest trying to find my way back home but with little success. Suddenly, I heard a menacing sound of men walking and realized that I was being hunted. In the dream I recall thinking that my parents used to tell me stories of running from the Nazis through the forests of Europe trying to escape capture. I then came to a river that I could not cross because it was full of raging water, like Moses at the Red Sea. I nevertheless built a bridge to get to the other side of the river but when I looked downward, I noticed that the river was not full of raging water, but raging shit. I was terrified that I would fall into the shit river and die. I asked God to help me but there was no answer. I then woke up in a sweat.

Being the methodical electrical engineer Avi associated to the dream, scene by scene. He said that him wandering in the forest reminded him of his parents who were on the run for many years before they were apprehended by the Nazis. Avi said that he still felt guilty for what his parents had gone through and he was complaining about a little back pain! He linked the menacing men hunting him to the Nazis who hunted his parents and other Jews during the Holocaust. It also made him think about all of the people who were out to get him because he was a perfectionist at work and in his friendships. As for the river, Avi said that he once nearly drowned in a river as a young man and the anxiety and fear he felt at the river called to mind his near dying childhood experience. As to the bridge, Avi said that he often felt estranged from people and did not know how to bridge the distance between him and friends and colleagues, sometimes even his wife and children. That the raging river turned into a raging river of shit was equated with the intense anger he felt at people who tried to pass off their "shitty" work as something worthwhile. Feeling so angry also made him feel like shit as it messed up his orderly way of being-in-the-world and made him feel so out of control as opposed to his usual meticulous way of thinking and doing. He also said that the shitty river reflected his fear of getting sick, old and dying and ending up as fertilizer for the worms as he described it (Avi was obsessed with dying and often wondered what would happen to him after he dies). In addition, he reflected on his worry that not only would he end up as fertilizer but that everything he worked on would end up as shit as he got older and less effective.

For our purposes, what is important in this dream and associations is the way that excrement is used as a symbol: of Avi's anger at others and wish to aggress them; and his fear of decrepitude, ageing and dying. The power of the image of the excremental river is possibly the key to understanding this dream. It symbolizes all that is most negative, in terms of both physical and feeling states in the suffering dreamer.

Vignette Two

Larry, age 34, a lapsed Catholic as he called himself, worked in computer technology for a start up company. He was single though living with a woman for about a year in an apartment on the upper West side of Manhattan. Larry came to me because he was unreasonably angry at his boss who did not promote him but rather gave the promotion to an admittedly more qualified colleague. Larry felt very competitive with his colleagues and for that matter, with anyone he came in contact with. He went to an Ivy league university and was used to being treated as special by others, including his parents who he felt often lived through his financial success (they were both elementary school teachers). Larry could be very obnoxious in session, often trying to better me, just as he was hyper critical of anything I said that he regarded as ill-conceived. In the transference, I was viewed as either a benign father figure or a person he was envious of and in rivalry with. Below is Larry's urination dream.

> I dreamt that I was playing in Major League baseball for the Yankees, my favorite team. I had been up to bat twice and got hits, a single and a double. When I got up to the plate the third time, the audience cheered me on because the bases were loaded and we were down one run and it was the bottom of the ninth inning with two outs. When I got up to bat, I felt a wave of anxiety that the pitcher intimidated me because he could throw fast balls that were really fast and maybe he would intentionally hit me. As I swung the bat instead of getting a hit, piss came out of the bat like a squirt gun. The crowd booed me and I struck out because my bat could not hit properly given that it spouted piss.

Larry associated to the dream as follows. He said that despite his financial success he felt like a failure in his own eyes especially when he compared himself to other's his age. He always wanted to be a professional baseball player but was not nearly good enough to play Major league baseball. What troubled Larry most about the dream was that he let down his team and struck out. He felt ashamed for his inadequacy. As for the fast ball pitcher Larry said he often felt intimidated by his colleagues who he though was better at the job than he was. Larry also mentioned that as a child he was on the smaller side compared to his friends and was sometimes teased. Larry thought the urine spouting baseball bat was a bizarre image. It was an image that evoked deep feelings of shame and humiliation at having a penis that didn't work properly like a leaking baseball bat. He related it to the fact that he often felt that he was not what he seemed to be, that appearance and reality did not mesh. Instead, he said he was like a little kid that was peeing himself, especially compared to his more successful colleagues and friends, success being measured only by income and acquisitions.

What is important about this dream is the way urine is symbolically used to signify Larry's competitive wishes on one hand, and his feelings of inadequacy, if not castration on the other hand. Larry acknowledged to me that he often put up a bravado front to people, even exaggerating his accomplishments so that they would respect him more. This being said, the sad truth was that Larry felt like a little boy with a little impotent penis where squirting urine stood for all that was ineffective and inadequate about him.

Vignette Three

Mickey, age 17, was a junior in high school in an affluent suburban neighborhood. He came to me due to his under functioning in school (he failed a few subjects and barely got by on the others and was a "wise guy" in classes he hated), and he was oppositional and defiant at home, frequently getting into arguments with his parents, especially his rather dominating and controlling father. His father was a driven business man who was financially very successful. His mother was more nurturing than his father, but feeble in her attempts to control him. Mickey also smoked a lot of pot which his parents knew about but could not stop him from doing after school and on weekends when he went out with his friends. When Mickey was in his room, most of the time he was gaming, Minecraft Dungeons being his favorite game, or talking to his friends on his cell phone. When I met Mickey, he was considering applying to a four-year college though he appeared to be destined to go to a junior college, which he said he would not do. He was very bright and if he applied himself he could have got into a first-class university. Mickey agreed to see me because his parents bribed him by telling him they would buy him a car if he saw me and got his grades up to a "B" average. I saw Mickey twice a week for two years. In the transference I was Mickey's protector having got his parents and school officials off his back. He viewed me as "on my side" in his war with adults. Mickey's dream is unique in that it includes reference to excrement and urination. Below is the dream.

> I dreamt that I was in English class which I hate. I hate the tea-cher, he is a lousy teacher, gives a lot of homework and is boring beyond belief. Anyway, in the dream I was called up to the front of the class to read a short section from Shakespeare which I had not prepared for, having not done my homework. I was afraid of being embarrassed and did not want to tell the teacher I did not prepare the section. I began to read the Shakespeare out loud and noticed that I felt like I was about to shit myself, being so nervous and embarrassed in front of the class. A few sentences into the reading the teacher looked angry and the kids in the class were laughing at me because they could smell the shit in my pants. I then woke up and the first thought I had was that I should have taken my dick out and sprayed them all with piss.

Not surprisingly, Mickey told me that the teacher reminded him of his father, because his father was always questioning him about school and the like and never appeared interested in what he was doing in his life that mattered to him. Mickey acknowledged that he loved his father because he was his father, but actually didn't like his father as a person. He could be very bossy, critical and controlling, calling to mind how Mickey viewed his English teacher, a man about his father's age and who was as much a "pain in the ass." Mickey believed that the tension he felt when reading (actually misreading the Shakespeare), also called to mind his father who made him feel inadequate when he would ask Mickey questions about current politics which Mickey had no interest in. Mickey felt that the shitting in class was like a little boy who has no control over his bowels which was really embarrassing to him. I agreed that this was a really embarrassing and humiliating episode but also wondered if it reflected his wish to shit all over the teacher/father figure, though he felt inhibited, actually afraid to do so. He agreed that his dream had to do with his father who gets him very mad most of the time, and he could see the desire to mess up his father in the "shittiest" way possible. As for the nervous embarrassment in front of the class, Mickey felt that the teacher had deliberately called on him with the intention of humiliating him, since the teacher probably knew that he did not prepare the Shakespeare as homework. This infuriated him as he felt the teacher aggressed against him by doing this and he wished he could punish him and get revenge on him for doing this. Mickey said that a part of him also felt embarrassed that he was such a lousy student but he did not know why he wouldn't put some effort into his studies, except that it was just too boring for him to properly attend to it.

The inadequacy that he was such a poor student evoked in him a feeling that he was damaged, his brain wasn't right. I commented that it seemed like the wish in the dream to spray everyone with urine was a wish to weaponize his penis to prove that he wasn't castrated, his brain/penis were not damaged.

References

Akhtar, S. (2009). *Comprehensive Dictionary of Psychoanalysis*. London: Karnac.

Des Pres, T. (1976). *The Survivor. An Anatomy of Life in the Death Camps*. Oxford: Oxford University Press.

Freud, S. (1925). Some psychical consequences of the anatomic distinction between the sexes. *The Standard Edition of the Complete Psychological Works of Sigmund Freud*, Trans J. Strachey with A. Freud assisted by A. Stratchey and A. Tyson, 24 volumes (1953–1974). London: Hogarth Press and the Institute of Psycho-Analysis, vol. 19, 241–258. (Henceforth *S.E.*).

Freud, S. (1909). Notes Upon a Case of Obsessional Neurosis, *S.E.* 10, 153–327.

Freud, S. (1905). Three essays on the theory of sexuality, *S.E.* 7, 135–243.

Freud, S. (1900). The Interpretation of Dreams. *S.E.* 4–5, 1–626.

Martins, I. (2022). Read the Latest Prostate Cancer News. https://prostatecancernewstoday.com/category/news-posts/feed/"[/vc_column][/vc_row] (retrieved 3/28/22).

Moore, B.E., & Fine, B. (1990). *Psychoanalytic Terms and Concepts*. New Haven: Yale University Press and the American Psychoanalytic Association.

Ricoeur, P. (1967). *The Symbolism of Evil*. Tr. Emerson Buchanan. New York: Harper & Rowe.

Scholz, M., & Blum, R.H.(2021). *Invasion of the Prostate Snatchers. An Essential Guide to Managing Prostate Cancer for Patients and their Families*. New York: Other Press.

Summers, S. (2022). The male urinary problem that won't just go away. https://healthcare.utah.edu/healthfeed/postings/2021/08/male-urinary-problems.php.

Vartolomei, L., Shariat, S.F. & Vartolomei, M.D. (2018). Psychotherapeutic Interventions of Targeting Prostate Cancer Patients: A Systematic Review of the Literature. *European Urology Oncology*, 1, 283–291.

Index

For Product Safety Concerns and Information please contact our EU
representative GPSR@taylorandfrancis.com
Taylor & Francis Verlag GmbH, Kaufingerstraße 24, 80331 München, Germany